LIGHT IN THE DARKNESS

Disabled Lives?

Missionaries of Charity
54A, Lower Circular Road
Calcutta-700016

Icu.   4/4/81

Dear Lady Lothian

Thank you for your kind letter.

I am sorry I am not able to write an article but I will pray for all those who are able to write what our Young Christians need. The joy of loving God and share this joy with all they meet and so become Instruments of Peace.

God bless you
M Teresa mc

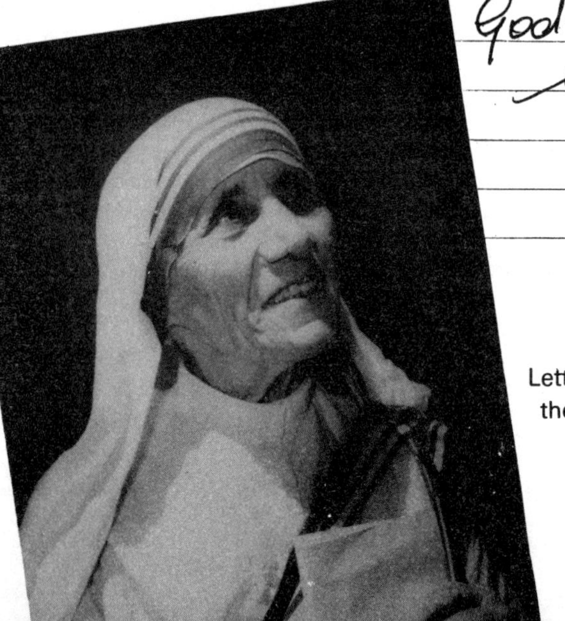

Letter sent to the President of
the Order of Christian Unity

LIGHT IN THE DARKNESS

Disabled Lives?

Papers on some contemporary medical problems.
Collected by The Medical Committee,
Order of Christian Unity.

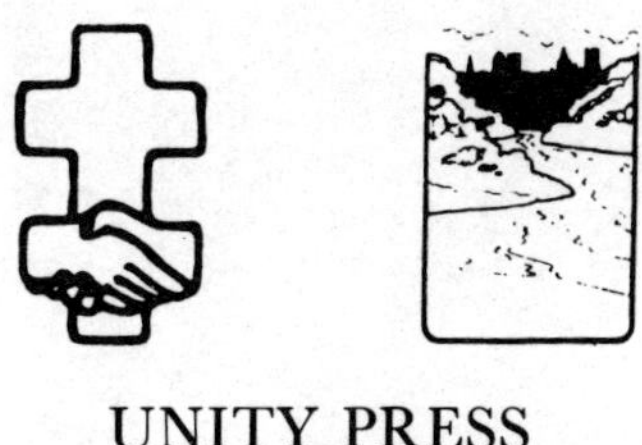

UNITY PRESS

MOWBRAY

ISBN 0 7289 0010 6

Cover Design by Julia Sappiro

Published for A. R. Mowbray & Co. Ltd. and Unity Press by Becket Publications

Also published:
Torn Lives?

Phototypeset by Cotswold Typesetting Ltd Gloucester
Printed in Great Britain by Biddles of Guildford

CONTENTS

PREFACE

Carl Marx said religion was the opium of the masses. Freud called it the Oedipus of the masses. Then Science took over and explained the awesome mystery of the Universe and split the tiny atom and released its horrendous energy, predicting that spiritual needs would wither away. Nevertheless modern man enters each decade with doubts and confusion, and a profound feeling that somewhere humanity, once again, has taken the wrong turning.

The purpose of this book is to look at part of the contemporary dilemma in spiritual and Christian terms—as well as in medical and scientific terms. Scientific publications tend to be 'statistical' or purely 'professional' usually with a hesitancy to express any inference, or offer guidance in the light of spiritual as well as physical experience.

We have therefore been fortunate to find from among many, a few leaders in both science and care for the community, who have had the courage to let their faith direct their commitment to medicine or community tasks. They take a stand against the tide of short-term fashions and in their quest to see beyond the immediate, have sought a deeper understanding of life so as to serve more completely those for whom they care.

In the introduction and the first part of the book, Sir John Peel, Professor Ian Donald, David Braine and Dr. Everett C. Koop write clearly argued and reasoned papers underlining some dilemmas of modern medicine and the stand they take as Christians in the light of their long and distinguished careers.

In the second part Pat Seed and John Steensma write of the potential in disability from their personal point of view as active Christians helping others also. Dr. Kingma gives a comprehensive and much needed account of the situation in developing countries. The third part contains papers by Dr. Scorer and Dr. West on the subject of dying and pain control giving a positive helpful approach. Group Captain Leonard Cheshire in the last paper writes of what true Christian compassion means in the light of the cross.

My thanks are due to Mother Teresa for the inspiration she gives us and her support in prayer during the preparation of the book. Thanks are also due to Dr. Ida B. Scudder, Emeritus Professor of Radiotherapy of the Christian Medical College, Vellore, for her valuable comments. The Marchioness of Lothian and Mr. Hartley Booth from the Order of Christian Unity have given continuous support and I am also grateful to Sir John Peel for his specific help together with the Medical Committee.

The book is produced by Unity Press and distributed by Mowbrays

Ltd, Oxford. We are most grateful to BCP Ltd and Julia Sappiro for
the cover design and frontispiece make-up.

DR. SETHURAJAN
Chairman, Medical Committee
Order of Christian Unity

INTRODUCTION
1. SOME DILEMMAS OF MODERN MEDICINE

Sir John Peel K.V.C.O. D.M. F.R.C.O.G. F.R.I.P. F.R.C.S.

In a recent article on the dangers to freedom in our society, Lord Chalfont wrote of "a deadly virus which has brought about a progressive decay of our national spirit, which often takes the form of contempt for anything which contains a suggestion of authority, tradition and dignity". He goes on to list the police, the judiciary, the monarchy and parliament as current objects of derision, and details many areas where standards have fallen steadily away with the consequent detestation of excellence and the elevation of mediocrity. In this climate of opinion, it would be surprising if the profession of medicine were to have escaped criticism and in fact it has been under such criticism and even attack from several different quarters and for a number of quite different reasons within recent years.

Progress versus Traditional Values

Many would agree that in previous generations doctors have tended to be too authoritarian. This was however, based upon knowledge, training and experience and tempered with a genuine caring for the welfare of the patient, which is not always apparent today. Within the profession itself, changing attitudes have been emerging. This is in many respects a good thing but I have been saddened to hear that some contemporary leaders of the profession have followed the permissive trend, abandoned their vitally important advisory roles and have stated publicly that doctors are not concerned with morals, that medical ethics are a matter of fashion, that, for example, it does not matter if schoolgirls become pregnant so long as they present themselves early for abortion, or that the incurable should be encouraged towards self destruction. These may not be majority views, and in a democracy minorities are given every encouragement to make their particular point of view. But the risk to democracy is apparent when the "pros" and the "antis" make their points of view more and more vociferously and sometimes violently. The more extreme the "pros" become, the more vigorous the "antis" emerge and majority decisions are constantly under threat, and general stability undermined. Uncontrolled "demos" have destroyed civilisations in the past, and history has a habit of repeating itself. In this climate of behaviour, are there any dangers for patients and doctors? is a question that must be answered in the affirmative. The ethos of medical practice has been based upon the principles of the Hippocratic tradition, which though established well before the birth of Christ, is in essence in complete harmony with the Christian concept of man, made in the image of God.

Respect for human life and concern for the patient's welfare as an individual are the cornerstones of medical practice. Religion and medicine have always been close, sometimes intimate bedfellows. Faith in the priest and faith in the doctor, have supported so many in their concern for their spiritual and bodily welfare.

In our modern materialistic world these faiths are becoming steadily eroded in the minds of the public whilst on the professional side there has been an unprecedented expansion of science and technology. The entry of the state as the major financial controller and the monopoly employer of doctors, adds a further item into the equation of the so called doctor/patient relationship.

Health, Ill-Health and Social Conditions

Some 15 years ago I wrote warning of what I saw as serious problems ahead for medicine, as doctors were more and more dividing themselves into two streams. On the one hand are those with a collectivist view of the doctors' role in society, concerned with the health of the community in terms of the cost effectiveness of the services provided, with prevention rather than cure as their motto; while on the other are the scientists, who regardless of cost, are concerned primarily with unravelling the intricacies of the human body as a fascinating piece of machinery. Both clearly have their place, but meanwhile the individual sick patient is all too often getting a raw deal. The growth of consumerism, pseudo education of the public, often aided and abetted by the media, together with the expansion of trades unionism into the hospital environment, has compounded the problems and helped to create an atmosphere of perplexity, anxiety and even hostility amongst all the members of the caring professions, as well as among the general public.

Many of these problems are highlighted in the recent series of Reith Lectures by Ian Kennedy. He chose the emotive title "Unmasking Medicine". I found these lectures interesting, even arresting, but a curious mixture of statements based on inaccurate information, interpretations and opinions presented as facts, and yet criticisms which must be taken seriously because they are amply justified.

The concept that much of the illness with which doctors have to cope in modern society is due to social and political factors, is of course true, but it is only half of the truth. To argue that doctors should do more to prevent rather than to attempt to cure such illness is to endow them with responsibilities for which they have not been trained. Doctors have known and emphasised time and again that health and ill health are closely related to social conditions, but to raise the standard of living of the poorer classes in society is surely outside the capabilities of the medical profession. To accuse doctors of being uninterested in prevention is unfair. They have in fact made enormous contributions to the prevention of many of the epidemic and communicable diseases, to improvements in maternal and perinatal mortality and morbidity and the journals are full of articles dealing with the best way of preventing this or that disability or disorder. Of course better housing, better nutrition, better sanitation have played a vital role but the two aspects of prevention are complimentary and multi-disciplinary.

Medicine and Behavioural Problems

Today there are different problems in relation to prevention. More and more of a doctor's time is taken up with disorders—illnesses and diseases as well as psychological disturbances—that have been created by deviations of behaviour. Such deviations are of course not new and human frailties have always been with us, but there are many new ones on the scene today, and doctors have not been lacking in their concern about them. A few examples suffice to emphasise the problem: Cigarette smoking is known to be related to lung cancer, bronchitis and heart disease. The abuse of drugs including alcohol, drunken driving, sexual promiscuity resulting in venereal diseases, unwanted pregnancies, abortion and degeneration of family life, are all on the increase. How are they to be prevented? I think by education at a personal level and more importantly the restoration of a greater sense of responsibility in the individual and acceptance of the need for higher standards of moral and ethical personal behaviour. Sadly, education is a very slow process. Experience shows that there is a very poor correlation between knowledge and education on the one hand, and motivation on the other. We know that cancer of the cervix in women could be almost entirely prevented by regular screening. It is not lack of knowledge, not lack of education, lack of facilities or services, that prevents the goal from being achieved; it is largely lack of motivation.

Control of Technological Advance

The rapid growth of scientific, academic and technological medicine during the last two or three decades has been remarkable and it would appear unreasonable in the extreme to be critical of this in any way. Enormous benefits have accrued to individual patients. It has become possible to do all sorts of things which were impossible before. But because you can do something does not mean that you should necessarily do it. The media, by highlighting every new scientific development in medicine long before the benefits can be universally applied, tends to create dissatisfaction in a society where the welfare state has raised expectations far beyond what the state can provide. Take for example embryo transfer—the so called "test tube baby". It is now possible under very special circumstances, to take the ovum from a woman, fertilise it by male sperm in vitro and then transfer the fertilised ovum into the uterus where it may grow and develop as normal. A marvellous scientific achievement—yes, but there will inevitably be those who will abuse this facility and how are doctors to avoid such abuses: for example the bribing of a surrogate mother?

Artificial insemination with donor semen has long been possible and now increasingly practised but again it needs little imagination to foresee the risks involved—moral and legal as well as physical, without a rigid code of practice. Transplant surgery grows from strength to strength, but here again some control is needed, but who should exercise that control? There are many other similar developments in scientific medicine which raise two other very vital considerations. In the first place, within a nationalised health service, considerations of cost and priorities are of prime importance, and herein rests a further dilemma for the doctor, concerned as he or she is with the individual patient. Should priority be given to the effective treatment of the common ailments which, while not serious to life, are incapacitating, or to the more sophisticated and elaborate treatments which may not in the end be completely effective? How far should resources be allocated to more trivial and sometimes purely aesthetic conditions, if it means depriving the handicapped or old? How far should resources be allocated to preventive measures at the expense of more immediate curative medicine? At present we are endeavouring to do all things and inevitably, failing in some degree all along the line.

Dispensable Life

Paradoxically much of the new technology is being successful in salvaging lives that would otherwise be lost, and thereby actually increasing the cost to society at large. This raises the most serious moral dilemma of all.

The numbers of those we may call the unwanted—unwanted by society and often by the family are ever increasing. By our abortion law we have decided that the unwanted foetus is disposable, even if it is unwanted for purely trivial reasons. We have therefore set our feet on a very slippery slope for reasons purely of convenience.

Next comes the congenitally abnormal neonate, the incurably ill, the mentally disordered and the senile. When the abortion act was passed in 1967 this warning was plainly spelt out but ignored and so we now have pressures for what is euphemistically referred to as Euthanasia—but in plain English—killing. If society wants these abominations, are doctors to be pressurised into acting as the agents?

The need for medical ethics is paramount, because if doctors are forced to go against any principle to which they adhere as right, then not only is medicine made the poorer but ethical behaviour in general must suffer. It is interesting that the World Medical Association will have before it later this year, a draft declaration on the right of the patient, which includes among other things, *the right to be cared for by a physician who is free in his clinical and ethical judgements.*

The Effects of Legislation

In spite of the fact that it is usually claimed that legislation cannot affect behaviour there are abundant examples of how legislation does affect attitudes both in doctors and in the public.

In our pluralistic society, we have seen a relaxation of many fundamental moral codes, often given official approval by equally permissive legislation based on such plausible fallacies as, crime will go away once you improve social environment; venereal disease and promiscuity will disappear if only people become better educated and if our youth receive sex education.

Distorted Objectives

Prior to the introduction of the Abortion Act in 1967, the majority of doctors were totally opposed to the form in which it was introduced. Within a few years, most of the profession has forgotten its moral principles and capitulated to further demand. The primary reasons given for its introduction were to reduce illegitimacy and avoid all the social and family problems created by large families, especially in the poorer classes. It was however obvious that the effect of the legislation in the form in which it was planned would have inevitably led to a large increase in unwanted pregnancies in young girls, and this is precisely what has happened. From a few hundreds before the 1967 legislation, the number of teenage pregnancies has grown to 75,000 in 1979 of which 10,000 were in children under the age of sixteen. Obviously the legislation is not the only causative factor in this sorry state of affairs, but there is little doubt that it has contributed. And so slow are we to learn lessons from experience, that we now have more and more clamouring for contraceptives freely available on request at any age, more, and more sex education, and the abolition of the age of consent! If the aim of sex education is to reduce the incidence of

5

illegitimacy, unwanted pregnancy, promiscuity and venereal infections in young people, then as currently practised it can claim remarkably little success. If doctors show reluctance to participate in furthering such practices, to what extent will they be further pressurised by the powers that be, by consumers and the other pressure groups?

The Allocation of Resources

The second criticism levelled at the medical profession by the Reith Lecturer and others who agree with him, is that too much of the national resources are being devoted to the expansion of academic medicine, which is always expensive in both manpower and equipment.

I must confess to having some sympathy with this criticism. We must not, and indeed should not, impede the progress of medical knowledge and we must do all we can to keep the frontiers of medical progress moving forwards. But is academic medicine too involved in research? It is given to few to acquire the aptitude to make real and significant contributions to new knowledge, if indeed such aptitude can ever be acquired if it is not inborn. I have always felt that there is far too much overlap and reduplication in the research programmes of different academic units and a greater need for co-operation and collaboration to prevent such overlap. Further, because of the increasing use of medicines and apparatus in the wards of our hospitals, many patients complain of a lack of personal interest in themselves as people, rather than in their disease, by those who are attending them. I can understand and sympathise.

Who is to Control Medicine?

Ian Kennedy began his lectures by claiming that "We must become masters of medicine and not its servants"—but who are "We"? We are in a society where consensus becomes more and more difficult to achieve. Some of "us" want more prevention, some of "us" want more cure. Some of "us" want the abolition of private medicine, while some of "us" want more of it. Some of "us" want to expand the facilities for free abortions, some of "us" want them restricted. Some of "us" want better facilities to treat our common ailments—our hips and our hernias, some of "us" want more intensive care units after our coronaries and our strokes—and so on, *ad infinitum*.

One of the difficulties that doctors have in the whole field of ethics is that morality is about absolutes—the value of human life is infinite. Doctors on the other hand are all the time having to make decisions based on the relative—the comparative effectiveness of different procedures, safety and risks of alternatives. Furthermore they have to operate within the contemporary mores of society, and within the social and political climate of the times.

Minority pressure groups, claiming to speak on behalf of the public, abound, and much of their actions impinge on the practice of medicine. In a society which lays so much store by material welfare one senses a desire to eliminate the increasing numbers of the unwanted and doctors are called upon to act as the technical agents.

Medical Technician versus Doctor to Individuals

The doctor's primary concern is for the welfare of the patient and the Christian doctor is always mindful of the great injunction of the Christian faith "To love thy neighbour as thyself." But how does he, the doctor, do just that when the patient's demands for what he considers to be in his own interest, conflict with the basic principles of his own moral code?

The twentieth century is as full of "prisoners of conscience", so significantly portrayed in the magnificent new east window in Salisbury Cathedral, as previous centuries have been—only the form is different. The Christian doctor in our modern secular society is so often rowing against the tide of public opinion.

Some of our modern doctors espouse the role of the technician and declare that morals are no concern of theirs. It is easier that way. In our heart of hearts what every one of us wants is, that when we are really ill, with perhaps a fever, pain or other symptoms, we want the services of a kindly doctor who knows how to diagnose our illness, explain its causes and apply the appropriate treatment with skill and consideration for us as individuals. In reality this is what the practice of medicine is all about.

Dr. Burkitt wrote some years ago, "In the whole approach to the urgent problems of medical ethics we can scarcely do better than adopt the words of a well known hymn as our prayer for the right attitude.

> May the mind of Christ my Saviour
> Live in me from day to day.
> By his love and power, controlling
> All I do and say.".

Part 1
A Positive Approach to Life

2. PREVENTING HANDICAP

Professor Ian Donald C.B.E. M.D. F.R.C.O.G. F.R.C.S. Hon. F.A.O.G.

I

Antenatal care and good supervision in labour are making very significant contributions to child welfare. But abortion has nothing to do with research, except where undertaken because of scientifically proven handicap whereby detailed tissue examination may yield important information. Otherwise it is not a part of the research worker's commitment.

Eugenics is a political, not a medical issue and must in no way be confused with the objectives of genuine research bodies interested in the baby, both before as well as after its birth.

I could spend far more time on what I have not done than on what I have done. It is to my engineering friends in Glasgow and Edinburgh in Nuclear Enterprises that the real credit is due. I only set out to solve some common clinical problems. I used an established metallurgical technique with surprisingly gratifying results, later improved by display methods developed in radar and later still in the case of grey-scaling, by the principle of scan conversion derived from radio technology. The ability which all this provided to study the developing baby *in utero* without disturbing it is now a matter of history but these same babies are tomorrow's citizens and heritage.

According to *The Lancet* in 1977, there were 33,000 badly handicapped children in the United Kingdom and a further 100,000 moderately so. We should no longer think of life's span as being from the cradle to the grave but rather from conception. There is after all a genetic continuum in all of us, each one testifies to the wonder of creation—the miracle of life.

I myself, like so many fortunate ones, have not been put to the test of having a crippled child like other parents, and I wonder if I would match up to it as they so often do with united families and dedicated workers, who seek to share the good fortune of their health with those whose lives would otherwise be meaningless.

If man was made in God's image, then let us recognise the faults in our creation which occasionally spoil that image.

Genetic science is new but is itself pregnant with possibilities forever accelerating research. At least, like physics, it is blessed with accuracy and objectivity and not without a certain humility which all who are concerned with the everyday miracle of human reproduction must acknowledge.

The day may yet come when we regard cerebral palsy, for example, and related handicaps as preventable and this would involve not only better ante and intrapartum[1] care, but a fuller knowledge of the genetic contribution to the problem and what, if anything, could be done about it.

The birth of a handicapped child[2] automatically raises two questions in the minds of the affected family. One is what to do about it and the other is why it should have happened. The first calls for treatment, however difficult, and the second for research which may be even more challenging.

The appalling infant mortality of a century ago with its even greater associated infant morbidity can no longer be accepted with devout resignation any more than disease which advanced medical care can now remedy. The trouble about child handicap, including mental retardation, is that here we have hardly yet begun. Many are the genetic secrets and their mechanisms yet to be prized open by further research.

No doctor can foresee what the future may hold in store for the handicapped child, or his parents, and how they may react. What is urgent is that every remedial method, both by the Government, by research bodies and by society as a whole should be invoked in helping to share the load with which the parents may be faced. How difficult for the gynaecologist to make a life or death decision when faced with a proven handicap as a result of antenatal screening. How presumptuous to assess how adequately or otherwise the family will adjust to the tragedy when it occurs. The remedial help which a caring society can muster can work wonders with the skilled help of neurosurgeons, physiotherapists, speech and occupational therapists and the like.

Good can indeed come out of evil and there are many centres whose work should be more widely known and assisted. The Central Remedial Clinic in Dublin, which I know, started in 1951 simply to cope with cases of paralysis from poliomyelitis. Now it copes on a national scale with all manner of disabling conditions in young people. Its number includes almost 800 children with cerebral palsy and 66 with spina bifida; 160 children are attending the school and over 100 are now sufficiently grown up and trained to work in the workshop.

I saw a film in Yugoslavia of children with cerebral palsy and barely able to stand, let alone walk, learning with special help to ski in 3 days better than I could ever hope to.

In this country too, in places such as the Hester Adrian Research Centre in the University of Manchester, it is reckoned that the potential of the mentally handicapped has hitherto been seriously underestimated and consequently neglected. In their management of Down's Syndrome[3] for example, beginning as soon as possible after birth they have shown a remarkable improvement in I.Q. from just over 40 to over 60 if home based care is begun in the first 6 months of life. They thus prevent developmental delay which is cumulative and leads to what is called secondary handicap through neglect of the first. These results have been further confirmed in 40 cases of Down's Syndrome in the Child Development Centre in Memphis, Tennessee.

All this very much involves the obstetrician and paediatrician and may affect the mother's whole attitude to her tragic problem.

The founder of a centre set up in Athens in 1972 told me that in Greece most parents remain uninformed, alone and "unassisted".

All over the world the problem of foetal handicap challenges the creative magic of compassion. A democratic state exists to serve its citizens, even the least of them, not the other way round.

There are so many dozens of different hereditary diseases requiring different screening methods that no one laboratory could hope to cope. Yet there are those whose attitude towards research is one of "Stop—enough is enough". Only the ignorant and the prejudiced can take such a view. Just consider the danger of babies being aborted because of the possibility, not even the certainty, of disablement: for example from rubella in early pregnancy without serological proof of the need for it. This is now universally available by laboratory technology.

Technology often outstrips clinical acceptability, but even so there is great need to improve the geneticists' therapeutic weapons which are restricted to genetic counselling which may be negative, the recommendation to terminate pregnancy which is even more so, or genetically controlled reproduction as in the veterinary world.

I myself, would not like to feel that I had contributed to a Huxleyan *Brave New World* Society.

Research to neutralise harmful genetic influences is badly needed. Few would from choice subscribe to a method of coping with handicap by liquidating the victim, after birth or before. Better methods must be found.

My innate abhorrence of abortion without scientific or medical indication of the need for it is well known and it is with great sadness that I recognise that the gynaecologist of tomorrow, or even today, is likely to be called upon to destroy more human life than he can hope to save in a clinical lifetime. It is a unique situation unparalleled in any other branch of medicine. So far at least it has not extended to geriatric medicine nor psychiatry.

In the United Kingdom now about 120,000 abortions are notified to the authorities each year. To this murderous score should be added an unknown number of abortions not so notified. Obviously abortion never saved a single baby's life, although occasionally, an aborted foetus survives for a time in spite of what was intended for it. As for saving a mother's life by abortion, this is now a matter of rare necessity thanks to modern medical care. Admittedly the gynaecologist is also concerned in other fields such as infertility, sterilisation, family planning, endocrinology and certain reparative procedures, none of which can be classed as life-saving, apart from occasional cases of haemorrhage from various causes. Even those of us who have been concerned with gynaecological cancer reckon more in terms of prolonging life than actually saving it.

It is one of the contradictory anomalies of this age that we have on the one hand perinatologists (specialists in baby care during and immediately after birth) seeking with dramatic success, I might say, to salvage the high risk cases and endless approaches are made to the problems of infertility in couples of poor reproductive performance, versus the almost unlimited abortion, literally by the hundred thousand, of the genetically sound but socially unwelcome future citizens. We thus yield to the pressures of Western materialism, in a world that has not only lost its sense but its sensibility.

Aborting the handicapped can actually increase selectively the gene pool of disease carriers, particularly for example in cases of sex-linkage, thereby transferring the problem from this generation to the next. The classic example is haemophilia, handed down from Queen Victoria to some of the male members of the royal families of Europe, including particularly the only son and heir of Czar Nicholas. So numerous are the harmful genes for which each one of us is fortunately heterozygous,[4] that no screening coverage, however universal, could ever hope, except in a very few instances to abolish the problem of the handicapped or crippled child who, like the poor, will always be with us, though its type and emphasis may change.

Selective abortion may seem an easy and expedient way out of an individual situation but is a short-sighted policy. It does not even go halfway towards solving the problem. I need hardly remind you that if the present day casual attitude towards abortion in general had operated 30 years ago, the wonders of treatment and prevention in Rh haemolytic disease[5] might never have come about. It would have been simpler in those days to abort than go to the modern extravagant lengths of exchange transfusion, intra-uterine transfusion and the prophylactic preparation and use of modern immunoglobulin in susceptible patients identified immediately after delivery. As it is, thanks to the research teams of such men as Liley and Clarke, the problem may be 90% eliminated from obstetric practice within the next decade. Certain inborn metabolic disorders likewise.

The decision to deny the right to life of the physically and mentally handicapped, diagnosed before birth, is one which has to be taken by the involved parents and their thoughtful doctor. It is not for us to judge but let us not cheapen that decision by confusing it with the prevalent philosophy of wholesale abortion simply on the grounds of threatened social inconvenience, thereby becoming, in the words of Valerie Riches of the Responsible Society, "technical weathercocks".

When faced however, with the certainty of deprivation in the unborn but handicapped child, the matter becomes challenging indeed. How difficult to distinguish between the sadness or tragedy of the families involved and the possibility that the affected child itself may be helped to find life worth living. All the greater therefore, is our responsibility to assist with remedial research.

Mid-trimester abortion unfortunately, is a traumatic business for the patient both physically and psychologically. Our dislike of abortion can be compared with our civilised dislike of capital punishment, euthanasia, flogging and torture. It is not just the victim for whom we are concerned, it is the general brutalising effect they have on those who carry them out, assist, witness or vicariously encourage them, including the public, eager for every scrap of news: for example, of an execution. As the French said, "Nous sommes tous meurtriers."[6]

Unless the diagnosis of foetal handicap stimulates research in managing it or at least mitigating its worst effects, the danger of screening, resulting in a sort of witch hunt to eliminate the threatened survivors is likely to provoke a measure of hostility in a public already suspicious, and rightly so, of authoritarian technology. Multiplication of screening tests, even assuming 100% accuracy, can only multiply the doubt and anxieties of countless women unnecessarily, and they must be applied with discriminating care.

There is a difference between "pity" and "compassion". When we talk of putting an old person, or a dog, or a handicapped child out of an existence which we ourselves see as miserable, we are often acting out of pity; perhaps more for ourselves than the sufferer. Compassion is altogether different and calls for constructive effort and all the love and costly care that good people can provide. Funds for such research are unlikely to come tumbling in exactly from Government departments interested in cutting costs (a process made futile by an ever-increasing bureaucracy). To such, abortion may seem the cheapest and simplest way out of a social responsibility. In fact, a civilised society such as ours is alleged to be, cannot accept such a philosophy, but itself should make more research available.

II

Does belief in Christ help in one's clinical practice and decision making? It may surprise you to learn that although it may make decisions clear enough, in practice it may provide endless trouble and problems for the believer.

In this respect, gynaecology is a particularly vulnerable branch of medicine. In gynaecology it is easy enough to know what is right but this may involve swimming against the tide today.

I need only mention the subject of abortion without a proper and honest reason. As you may know, I have consistently campaigned against the wanton liberal policy of abortion on demand, or "request", however you like to phrase it. Like so many of my profession I feel that to carry out any surgical procedure on a patient without a good reason is highly unethical; and when that operation involves the sacrifice and destruction of the life of another it is indefensible to regard the matter as trivial.

I don't think that one can or should be an absolutist in the matter of abortion. A value judgement, that hateful phrase, must not be shirked. One's Christian outlook inevitably influences that judgement. Would Christ Himself, who did so much to heal others of their afflictions, have supplied abortion on demand? I think not. Where the mother's health or life are at severe hazard there is really no problem, since one might lose both. These cases are now rare, thanks to the advances in medical care which make it possible to save both; in fact in many cases of severe heart disease in the mother it is often possible to get her through her pregnancy and delivery fitter than she was before.

The problem really comes when confronted with serious foetal abnormality, the likelihood of which can now be so often foreseen, thanks to modern diagnostic aids. At what point does one decide whether an unborn child has got the expectation of a life worth living, bearing in mind that to conserve such a pregnancy may increase the hazards to the mother meanwhile?

There are all degrees of abnormality and handicap, from the very severe which may be incompatible with eventual survival, to genetic or congenital disorders which, though distressing particularly to the parents, may still leave the baby with the chance of a happy and useful life. Sometimes such diseases are treatable after birth but more often they are not. Unfortunately this applies particularly to disorders associated with mental handicap—surely every pregnant woman's greatest dread.

Where do you place the cut-off point, bearing in mind the room for error which dogs all clinical judgement? When in doubt, do nowt is a good obstetrical principle which I have seldom had cause to regret. My own personal cut-off point is when it is cast iron clear that the child will be so mentally defective as to be incapable of spiritual development, and there are diseases in which this terrible prognosis can be made with certainty. I cannot believe that God is either to blame or wishes to inflict such tragedy on parents however loving. It would be so much simpler never to have made the ugly discovery in the first place and I have had patients who made it quite clear that they would take what God had sent them and would never agree to termination of their pregnancy and this is a very welcome let-out for the doctor. No more antenatal diagnosis obviously.

Mercifully such cases are a very small proportion of the abortions which one is asked to carry out. You have to see it against the background of biological wastage which we now know to be very common in human pregnancy. Only a very small minority, the tip of the iceberg, get through to the end of pregnancy to emerge as seriously deformed or handicapped children.

The destruction of perfectly healthy unborn life in healthy women because of the great nuisance value foreseen, rightly or more usually wrongly, and as a means of long-stop contraception, because of failure or neglect, is something which one could never regard as God's work. Here one is at once in conflict with current opinion in today's changed world. How difficult for a Catholic now, or anyone with religious belief, to get on in gynaecology where these bristling problems abound.

Other ethical problems loom on the horizon of the gynaecologist. For instance Artificial Insemination donated in cases of proven male infertility. I fear, not without reason, that the practice may come in time to encourage selective stock breeding, as already in cattle, and may encroach upon the sacramental aspect of marriage about which Christ's teaching was clear and unequivocal.

Faith, the love of God and Redemption apply to us all. The professional standing of any one of us is of very secondary importance. Each of us can confess the King of Glory.

You might well ask how someone with my scientific background should have less difficulty, not more, in recognising that miracles, indeed all acts of God are possible. One has only to consider the nature of matter itself. Matter is not just a question of molecules, nor even of atoms. Atoms themselves are made up of differing electrical charges and as we now know can be both split and fused, given sufficient power.

There is more to a man's being and identity than a double helix, even though today it is more fashionable to think about chromosomes than about the Kingdom of Heaven. Faith itself requires built in opportunities for unbelief. It would not be a matter of Faith if proof were already available. Deny the existence of God and then you can and must deny the purpose of living. The only alternative is to regard one's life as a mere incidental accident in the course of a solar thermonuclear explosion—extended in our concept of time, but clearly trivial in terms of the universe.

It is, however, difficult and challenging to understand God. It is necessary to go back to the Old Testament to understand the all-powerful, creative and jealous God who would stand for no other gods. As Jesus himself said, "No man hath seen God at any time save only the Son." (JnI: 18) But we can all understand the vision of God made manifest in Christ. "In the beginning was the Word and the Word was with God and the Word was God"—"And the Word was made flesh and dwelt among us." (JnI: 1,14)

Surely, the point is do we or do we not believe in the purpose of life and the life hereafter? Jesus himself left us no room for doubt when, in the midst of his own agony, He said to the thief being crucified alongside him, "This day shalt thou be with Me in paradise."[7]

Of course miracles are possible. They are not to be disposed of by academic theologians as myths, however poetic. Deny one and you might as well deny the lot, deny the Resurrection and deny Christ himself. Alas there is a modern vogue of denigrating Christ, denying His divinity as well as His Resurrection. The devaluation of God appears to be an ingredient of much of today's philosophy. These arguments will die while the letters of Paul and the gospels will endure for hundreds of years yet to come. As Christ said, "Heaven and earth will pass away but my words will not pass away."[8] Remember John Bunyan's verse:

> "Who so beset him round with dismal stories,
> Do but themselves confound,
> His strength the more is
> Then fancies flee away, I'll care not what men say
> I'll labour night and day
> to be a pilgrim."

I love the motto of my University of Glasgow—Via, Veritas, Vita. The way, the truth and the life. And so it is very meet right and our bounden duty that we should at all times and in all places give thanks to Thee, Father almighty and everlasting God. Note that:- "At all times and in all places".

Notes

1. Before and during birth.
2. See also Dr. Koop's Paper p.27.
3. Commonly known as mongolism.
4. Carrying genes that are different from each other.
5. A condition that destroys red blood cells in the foetus or newborn.
6. Each one of us could be a murderer.
7. Luke 22:43.
8. Matt. 24:35.

3. WHY ABORTION?

David Braine

I wish to consider in as analytical a way as possible, deliberately avoiding emotion, what seems to me the primary question raised by this large-scale practice of abortion. This is the question whether or not abortion involves the taking of human life in essentially the same sense that killing a child the day after birth would do. One's answer to this question, one way or the other, is absolutely crucial. If a person did not think that abortion involved the taking of human life, he might very well still object to it for a variety of medical or other reasons, but the matter would no longer have the same gravity.

The key importance of this question can be high-lighted in the following ways:

Present Values in Society

If the foetus counts as having a human life *in the same sense as* the newborn child, then for most people in our society it will seem plain either: that one should never directly take its life at all, or: that one should only do this in a very limited number of special types of case. On the other hand, if it does not count as human life, then (rightly or wrongly) to very many people, in the present state of belief and attitudes in society, abortion will seem acceptable in a much wider range of cases.

The Effect on "Medical" Judgement

If the foetus counts as human life, it will no longer be possible to set a "medical" or "clinical" judgement in opposition to an "ethical" one. When a pregnant woman solicits the help of a doctor, the doctor may have only one "client", but he will have two "patients", in the sense of two individuals in his care. And, even if the foetus were not considered to have equal rights with the mother, still, if it counts as human life in the same sense as the newborn, it will have *some* rights, still make *some* call upon the doctor's care so that there are two "patients" not one. The question of what is "medically better" will not be the question of what is better for the mother alone, but of what is better for the mother and the child.

The Responsibility of the Law

If the foetus does not count as a human life in the same way as the newborn, then many will feel (rightly or wrongly) that the decision (right or wrong) whether or not to have an abortion should rest primarily with the mother, and that to think otherwise would be to impose one's own morality upon her. However, if the foetus is comparable with the newborn, then this argument does not get off the ground: the situation will be that of protecting the foetus or child from death as a result of the values or desires of others, a function which it is natural for the law to try to perform.

The Psychological Health of the Mother

On the one hand, if the mother who has had an abortion either seriously thinks or at some deep level (whether rationally or irrationally) feels that what has happened is the destruction of a child, then it would seem natural to expect that she will be much more liable to long-term distress than if she did not think or feel the matter in this way. And some people would raise the question whether, if she did not show any regret or distress while still thinking of abortion in this way, this might not be a sign of her being less human in some way; e.g., less capable of deep relationships and sympathy with other people. On the other hand, if she neither thinks nor feels the matter in this way, then it will be unsurprising if she is free from these long-term difficulties. Therefore: any adequate psychological research ought to take cognizance of what she thinks or feels the nature of abortion to have been, and in addition there is obviously a quite vital human question as to which is the *appropriate* way for her to think and to feel. On the one hand, if abortion is *not* comparable to destroying a child, then we would wish her to be quite free from these long-term difficulties. On the other hand, if abortion *is* comparable to child killing, then it would be quite wrong to lead her to seek an abortion, or to build up public pressure to grant her an abortion, or to base her psychological health, on the basis of a pretence that it is not comparable in this way.

Abortion Comparable with Infanticide or Contraception

The key question is, in effect, this: Is abortion comparable, as some say to infanticide, *or* is it more comparable to contraception? Both views are conscientiously held. The question is as to which is right, and this is not a political question, but very largely a factual one to which I now turn.

The newborn child is distinctively human in a biological sense, exhibiting features peculiar to the human species, not only in its genetic make-up, but also in its physical features and behaviour. Yet it does not yet exercise personality or rationality, but only has a potentiality for this exercise. It has a human life, then, in this sense that it is an individual biologically human organism, with the potential for rational or reflective activity and personal relationships later on as part of its nature. And in so far as the life of the child has value in itself, and not just because it would distress others for it to die, it is because it is human in this sense.

Evidently, this same organism with the same potential and the same value already existed in the womb before birth. The question is: How soon during pregnancy?

Clearly enough, the same organism with the same potential already existed before so-called "viability", whether by this one means the capacity to survive without special medical assistance, or whether one means the capacity to survive with the help of all available medical aid. The law of the U.K. in effect deems viability doubtful until 28 weeks,[1] and the Lane Report[2] recommends that this be changed to 24 weeks, but foetuses have in fact survived and so shown themselves viable with medical help before 20 weeks. Plainly, the viability of the foetus as ordinarily understood depends upon many things quite independent of how human it is, e.g., the previous nutrition of the mother; the strength of its heart; the skill and equipment of the medical profession, and its availability. Viability seems (in reason, even if not in the law of the U.K.) irrelevant to the human status or value of the life of the foetus—although it would be natural to suppose that it was very relevant to the duties of the mother, in that she would have more duty to continue bearing the child while its life absolutely depended on her, than after viability, when a premature delivery might often be justified.

And what seems to me sufficiently clear is that there is *no good reason for doubting* that the human organism, with human life in the sense I defined, in the same way as the newborn child, is already present before the eighth week after conception. At eight weeks indeed, the individual human being is not only established in an organised functioning bodily existence, capable of some movement, possessed of its main organs, and distinctively human in anatomy, with the frontal lobes of the brain already more developed than other mammals, but also even appears human in the general shape of its head and body. After that time, enormous development takes place, in size, in myelinization[3] and nervous communication and in the detailed organisation of the brain, but these developments continue even after birth. Perhaps it is worth noting that many mammals are born much sooner after the stage man reaches at seven weeks than man—the marsupials being an extreme case of this. Nothing in the study of mammals suggests that the times of birth and viability, so variable between the species, have any ontological significance for the status of a foetus: rather they have to do with size, nutritional arrangements, ecology, etc.

As to when, before this, human life actually begins, that is a more difficult question. Since the seventeenth century, the usual view has been that the individual human organism comes to existence at conception. However, there are rational grounds upon which this can sensibly (whether rightly or wrongly) be questioned. Thus, until about the 14th day, it is still possible for identical twinning to arise, so that someone might argue that the human individual only came into existence after such twinning ceased to be possible, and someone might associate the emergence of the individual with those developments (days 14–16) associated with the appearance of the primitive streak, which determine the emergence of an individual notochord[4] and central nervous system (days 17–19). Or someone might try to argue that until sometime during the key period in the development of the principal organ systems (say, days 18–30), the human organism is not established because not yet actually functioning as a unity within an environment clearly distinguishable from it. Or, again, I think much less plausibly, someone might argue that the proper functional unity of the human organism involved a functioning link between its principal parts and the central nervous system, a development which it is not clear has occurred before the seventh week, when generalised reflex movements begin to appear, as well as electrical activity in the brain.

I do not say that these arguments are right, but only that they are at least of the right sort, if the question is as to when the individual with human life in the sense I defined comes into proper existence: and the doubts they raise are set within very narrow bounds. Even if, from a philosophical point of view, in the present state of our biological knowledge (e.g., as to how far the developments in different parts of the embryo between days 20 and 30 are independent of each other, and how far induced from some core of already partly differentiated tissues, or as to how the functioning of the nervous system develops), it were arbitrary where to draw the line, this arbitrariness can be set within narrow limits, inside the first seven weeks. Inside that period, I see possible grounds for rational doubt as to how soon the human individual comes into proper existence: but *I see no grounds at all for drawing any line between the eighth week and some time appreciably after birth.*

Therefore, so far as I can bring reason to bear on this question, the only morally relevant differences between early infanticide and abortion (at least from the eighth week onwards) seem to me to lie in the greater distress to the mother, and greater degree of psychological realisation by a larger number of people of what is being done. So far as the taking of human life is concerned, they do not appear relevantly different.

Every case in which a mother seeks an abortion is fraught with human difficulty. Amidst this difficulty, some people will say that

abortion will still sometimes be justified, even if it is more comparable
to early infanticide than to contraception. And one sees the pressures
which can drive them to feel this.

Social Dependence on Abortion

But, through all this difficulty, what humanly one ought to insist
upon is the importance of thinking straight about the matter. Just as
one ought not to disguise from oneself the difficulties attending the
various alternatives to abortion, so also one ought not to disguise from
oneself what abortion involves. The much propagated ideas that
abortion is more comparable to contraception, and that what is
aborted is just some little formed tissues, or "part of the woman's
body", and not really human in such a way as to be compared to a
child, seem to run directly contrary to the facts, and to be entirely
without basis in either science or philosophy. And it seems quite wrong
to allow the acceptance of abortion by the public, or by mothers
sometimes influenced by public attitudes coming to seek it, to be built
up upon this kind of misinformation and pretence. It does not seem
right that the taking of human life, at any stage, should be made easier
in this sort of way. And, unwillingness to draw attention to facts which
suggest a comparability between the foetus from a quite early stage
and the newborn, or to let people think of them as comparable, is
doubly dangerous: it not only misleads people into an easier *acceptance*
of abortion as a solution for problems, but also leads to a neglect of the
social provisions for other solutions, and so to a greater *dependence* upon
abortion for their solution.

However, having insisted that in one's thinking about abortion one
should think straight, and recognise it as taking of human life, not just
in a verbal sense, but in such a way as to be more comparable to
infanticide than to contraception, there still remains the very serious
question, which some people will still wish to raise, as to whether
circumstances may not still sometimes justify and require it, and not
just in a few, but in many cases. And I want to consider this without
any appeal to religious insight.

Firstly, it may be asked, if the taking of life can be justified in war,
then why not in abortion? Here, three observations seem appropriate:

Those who think war can sometimes be right think of the killing in
war as an evil which is only justified as an extraordinary measure in
order to attain a just peace in which such killing does not occur, i.e.,
they think of killing as a grave evil, and as alien to the normal state
of society in peace.

Most human beings have thought that, other things being equal, it
is a graver evil to kill those who had not been wilfully doing

anything to one's harm ("innocent" people) than to kill people attacking one, and that the direct killing of children in war was either not justified at all (cf: German reprisal methods) or at least required more special reason.

Even if just war is in principle possible, it seems that very much or even most of the killing in most actual wars, even in wars it may have been right to fight, has been wrongful; the idea that in some special circumstances, grave reason may justify a limited war, has no tendency to justify the carnage which has actually occurred in war, or which necessarily occurs in total war.

Thus, the comparison with war, and consideration of the evils of war, would suggest that abortion on a large scale could never be justified, unless in the most extraordinary circumstances, and never as a normal incident of peace. .

Secondly it might be suggested that a utilitarian approach, valuing the greater secular happiness of the greatest number of already actually existing human beings (born or in the womb), might often justify abortion. Yet, upon examination, though the utilitarian might allow abortion in cases of highly probable severe handicap, and severe long-term unhappiness in the mother, he would still be very restrictive because the happiness of the child would still be of value to him—and there is no adequate evidence that illegitimate children, and children born into large families, even if sometimes delinquent, etc., have such an over-plus of unhappiness as usually to wish that they had not been born. And to justify the taking of an individual's life on the basis of rather vague and imponderable considerations and generalised statistics, is something many utilitarians would seek to avoid.

Thirdly, it might be suggested that what matters is only the happiness of those who at least are capable of being aware of wanting happiness, and that no wrong is done to a child or a foetus in taking its life, if it has not in this way entered the human "conscious community". Yet the problem is how to justify this view, which seems to restrict human duty in a rather arbitrary way, and in a way that runs contrary to the usual instinct or belief that we have more duty to the helpless than to those who can help or speak for themselves. There is always the danger amongst men that one will elevate a social contract between those with power or influence to help or harm each other into the status of a moral principle, leaving those with less influence out of account, as the Greeks left slaves out of account. Just as it seems right to insist upon the rights of women in relation to men, so it seems natural also to insist upon the rights of children in relation to adults in general.

Society and the state has the general duty to protect the human lives within its boundaries—and if my argument is correct then this will include children, even the newborn, and, along with the newborn, foetuses from a very early stage: i.e., from a stage earlier than the period (say 9 to 20 weeks) when most therapeutic abortions in practice occur. It will follow that the law should protect the foetus, as it protects others that cannot protect themselves, and permit abortion only for very limited and grave reasons.[5] And the primary means of controlling illegal abortions should not be by *imitating* them in terminating life, but by altering the attitudes and poor social facilities which press people into resorting to abortion, whether legal or illegal.

The argument I have presented does not depend upon any religious premises. It can be felt as forcefully by the secular humanist as by the believer. The notion of abortion as in any way a *normal* part of social or health service or population control policy, rather than as an exceptional measure to be considered only in very special circumstances, seems ultimately *alien* to any reflective kind of humanism, whether secular or religious.

Of course, to a person approaching the matter from the standpoint of Christian belief, if he works out the implication of his belief in a consistent way, the matter is liable to appear much clearer. If the child at birth is an individual human existent, whose existence will never come to an end, even in death, and which has the destiny of relationship with God, then reason will demand that the Christian consider the foetus, at least from a very early stage, in the same light. And, if Christ's Incarnation began in the womb, then so does the life of every man. Nor will it seem reasonable to any theist, whether Christian or not, who thinks of God as co-operating within creation, in his upholding all things in their existence and order, and therefore as co-operating in the making of each individual, directly to destroy a new person whom God has thus co-operated in establishing in existence, before he or she has come to the exercise of his or her personality: indeed, even if the individual is only properly established in existence after some weeks, it would still seem irreligious to destroy the pre-existing blueprint which came into existence at conception, even though this would not then be the taking of actual human life, and would not yet be properly comparable with infanticide.

But I do not here make appeal to these religious considerations, but only mention them in order to make clear how much my previous argument was independent of them, and depends only upon a generalised humanism which sees value in human life and in respect for other human lives, on the basis of a common human insight, without requiring appeal to religion to justify this.

I have not had space to discuss the important medical objections to abortion drawn from a consideration of the health of the mother and the effect upon later pregnancies, nor to discuss in detail the social, legal and statistical aspects of the problem. My main aim has instead been to establish what it seems to me ought, *if one is to be led by reason,* to be a fundamental datum in all these difficult discussions, namely that what is being talked about is the termination of a human life, not just in a verbal sense, but in such a way as to be comparable with taking the life of the newborn.

The key to the matter at the social level lies in public education. If society at large was made more fully aware of what is involved in abortion, and the state of human life in the womb, even early in pregnancy then there would be less pressure upon the medical profession to resort to abortion, and a greater drive to attend to other means, especially social means, to deal with the problems which give rise to this resort. It is difficult to see how the medical profession as a whole can have any reason for wishing to maintain the pressures which make them more dependent upon a practice, for which they themselves experience such revulsion. There seems no sense in allowing all the pressures they exert to be in one direction, towards the so called "liberal" stance. Yet the remedy is largely available in their own hands: by public education, to make the real nature of abortion more clear, instead of allowing the combination of their repute and their silence (in this regard) to leave this in doubt, disguised or unheeded; and, by willingness to co-operate with others, to encourage a different kind of social medicine to grow up, more consuming of time and attention, but less surgical in nature.

In the meantime, people conscientiously disagree on the matters, and those who disagree should have freedom effectively to influence each other by being together in groups, discussing and deciding the policies of departments, by being bound together in research teams whose results and mutual criticisms are published together, and by both having a role alongside each other in teaching those with a professional interest in the matter. And this is required even by the most traditional principles of liberalism.

Notes

1. This is stated in the abortion legislation of 1967.
2. 'The Working of the Abortion Act' 3 Vols. 1974, Cmd.No.5579.
3. Growth of nerve cell fibres.
4. This later becomes the individual spinal chord.
5. See Professor Donald's paper p.11.

4. PARENTS' PROBLEMS

*Dr. Everett C. Koop, M.D. Sc.D.(Med)**

In this paper I would like to point to some of the advantages to a family when a handicapped child is born to them.

The family, as the basis of our society, is not, after all, threatened so much by poverty, inadequate education and the lack of a more beneficent social planning government, as by the destruction of self giving love which is not compatible with the worship of the good things of this life. Deprivations when they exist can mold, knit and glue together the family structure which will survive and benefit as a result even in the face of cruel adversity. When a family is set only on obtaining more consumer goods, a handicapped child has little chance of being accepted and the birth will cause even more anguish.

Let me set the stage: When a family expects a baby they expect a bright-eyed chubby creature like the pictures on baby-food tins. Imagine the shock to a mother when she is told, however gently, that the baby has a congenital defect and immediate surgery is necessary if the baby is to survive. Even after this surgery she and her husband and any others in the family, will eventually discover that the baby will change all their very normal expectations about how the child can develop.

It is my belief that the baby—my patient—will do best in the heart of his family and that the shattered family can be rehabilitated. I know what can be accomplished in the habilitation of a child born less than perfect. I know what can be done with that child's family. I know that these children become loved and loving, that they are creative, and that their entrance into a family is frequently looked back upon in subsequent years as an extraordinarily positive experience.

I am aware that those who never had the privilege of working with handicapped children after the correction of a congenital defect think that the life of the child could obviously be nothing but unhappy and miserable. Yet it has been my constant experience that disability and unhappiness do not go hand in hand. The most unhappy children I have known have been completely normal. On the other hand, there is remarkable joy and happiness in the lives of most handicapped children; yet some have born burdens which I would have found difficult indeed to face. In the belief that when the family and the

* Adapted from a speech printed in *Human Life Review*, winter 1980, by kind permission of the author and the publishers of the journal.

handicapped child are given the proper support and guidance, they will all be better for the experience, it has been my lifelong practice to provide this support and guidance and I know it works.

For example, a young man, now in Graduate School was born without arms below the elbow and missing one leg below the knee. He was the victim of the prescription of thalidamide to his pregnant mother at the time of limb budding. With love and despite some confusion, there was a "happy ending" which is now only the beginning of that young man's productive life. Here is how the young man feels today: "I am very glad to be alive. I live a full, meaningful life. I have many friends and many things that I want to do in life. I think that the secret of living with a handicap is realising *who* you are—that you are a human being, somebody who is very special—looking at the things you can do in spite of your handicap, and maybe even through your handicap."

The arrival in a family of a child which might have died had it not been for skilled surgery presents the family with a crisis which is a threat to its unity and according to how the situation is coped with, indirectly to society in general.

Solutions and Non-Solutions

The alternative to surgical intervention in the case of a newborn with a serious congenital defect is to "allow" the baby to die. I have opposed this attitude more and more strenuously, over the last two years in particular, on the grounds that killing the patient in order to get rid of the defect has never been a part of responsible moral medical practice.

Although in more recent years I have become a specialist's specialist and my interests have been confined to those congenital anomalies incompatible with life but amenable to surgical correction, early on I was concerned with the management of cleft lips and palates, orthopaedic defects, spina bifida and its complications, congenital heart disease and major urological defects.

The physician responsible for the primary care of the family with a handicapped newborn child should act as overseer, guide and counsellor. In practice a family and their physician need to be in contact with a team that will do all it can to bring the pertinent agencies into contact with the family for their ultimate benefit. If a family has little support from the physician and no helpful information they are forced to work out what they need to know for themselves. In the U.S.A. their determination to keep the child at home will be met with hostility on all sides. Nevertheless, families who do succeed in adjusting to life with a handicapped child at home often form the nucleus of Foundations and Societies to help others.

The worst non-solution is to make financial resources (on the part of the family or the State) the main criterion for deciding whether to "allow" a newborn handicapped baby, who would die without surgery, to live. During a seminar in the United Kingdom which I was taking with the help of Professor Zachary, I was presented with this story. This is substantially what the questioner said: "I am a general practitioner in the National Health Service. Three years ago a daughter was born to us who had spina bifida and I was told she would die within 3 weeks. When a nurse told me she was being starved to death, I signed her out of the hospital against advice. She is now a bright, adorable, 3-year-old girl who is the light of our lives. However, she has an incontinent bladder and orthopaedic deformities which keep her from walking. Her spina bifida has never been repaired." We were able to tell her that the child could be made to walk in calipers and control her urine with an ileal bladder.[1]

'Allowing' a newborn handicapped child to die is a similar non-solution to the situation where the parent thinks that if he pays enough the physician must produce perfection! just as when he pays enough money for some 'consumer' product he gets the very best.

These attitudes are in contrast with a relationship between physician and patient where the patient can trust implicitly that he will receive the very best medical care available.

Computerised Support Data

After 35 years as the Surgeon-in-Chief of the oldest children's hospital in the western hemisphere, it is my hope that after the necessary adjustment, I can make available to physicians and parents a comprehensive service to take the sting out of managing a handicapped child. What I hope for is a national computerised service that could be accessed by physician or parent to provide for any handicapping diagnosis: the most competent diagnostic service closest to home, the closest competent therapeutic service, a list of all the available governmental and private agencies that could be of help to the parents and their children, and finally a readout of nearby parents with similar situations who have coped with the problem in the past.

If we could make this service available to parents and physicians alike, I think we would remove the terrible fear that exists, that the odds are too great against the handicapped child and his family to make any effort worthwhile. We could also gradually weaken the conviction that only perfect quality of life is life worth living.

Experience Cuts Costs

The first time that anything is done in Medicine will almost always be the most expensive time. As experience grows, as techniques improve, hospital care is shortened, rehabilitation is quicker, and the economic impact is far less.

For example: There is a major bony defect of the chest wall in children that requires correction if a child is not to be a cardiac cripple in adult life. During the operation in days gone by I used to transfuse these patients, post-operatively they were in oxygen tents, their hospitalisation consumed 3 weeks, and their return to normal activitiy was delayed for 3 months. Now, when in certain seasons of the year I do one of these every operating day, I never use a blood transfusion, post-operative oxygen is almost unheard of, hospitalisation varies from 3 to 7 days, and full activity is resumed 2 weeks after discharge. That is experience that cuts costs.

Ingenuity Can Restore a Patient to His Family

In the care that is absolutely essential to the surgical management of any congenital defect incompatible with life but amenable to surgical correction, there will be certain patients who become respirator dependent. As such they live in hospitals, they are extraordinarily expensive, and they are deprived of the nurture of the family because they cannot live at home.

It does not have to be this way. Taking our cue from a remarkable French experience in a northern suburb of Paris[2] we have now sent a number of respirator dependent patients home, we have had to revise the technology of their care, but in addition to the tremendous human benefits to the family and the patient, the cost has been cut from $600 (under £300) for care in a respiratory unit in the hospital to $40 (under £20) a day at home. As the numbers increase, I am confident that this cost can be reduced to $50 (£24) *a week*. Incidentally the process of weaning the child off the respirator is better accomplished in the loving environment at home than it is in the caring but nevertheless non-family atmosphere of the hospital.

The care of these children at home does not have to be done at the cost of government. Given enough patients at home on respirators, the French experience has shown that competitive free enterprise can deliver a superior service to patients and families than that provided by the government and can do it more cheaply.

This is only one instance where ingenuity can restore a child to his home and family at savings possibly through free enterprise, over the cost of governmental Medicine.

Beneficial side effects accrue to all of us from our attention to the care of the handicapped newborn: First of all, as the patient is benefited, so is his family. Secondly, the necessity for the special care required necessitates a new type of paraprofessional that makes the care of the next patient easier and cheaper but also has a spinoff for the care of patients with similar or related, if not identical, problems.

Finally, every so often there comes a time when the experience and sometimes the death of one child will provide untold benefits to other patients.

For example, a number of years ago a newborn child was operated upon in the children's hospital of Philadelphia and almost her entire bowel was found to be gangrenous; the unaffected bowel was not long enough to support life. In an institution aggressively seeking innovative procedures and trying desperately to push back the frontiers of pediatric surgery, one of my colleagues resected the gangrenous bowel and kept the child alive on total parenteral nutrition. She never ate by mouth; all her nutrition was supplied by vein. The hope was that a small bowel transplant would eventually be possible to restore this child to satisfactory existence. Before that technique could be achieved, the patient succumbed but until then she had been on total intravenous feedings, gaining weight and developing according to acceptable standards over a period of 400 days.

The cost was enormous. The patient died, but because she was the first to ever be maintained on total parenteral nutrition, medical science learned a great proportion of what it now knows about hyperalimentation or total parenteral nutrition from this one little girl.

It is without doubt one of the greatest medical advances of the past several decades. What we learned from that experience was intended for her own good and not for the good of society. But it did provide society with a now recognised nutritional technique which has saved the lives of thousands upon thousands of children and hundreds of thousands of adults around the world. In addition to that, hospital stays have been shortened, wounds have healed more quickly, rehabilitation has been possible sooner, and hitherto unmanageable situations like small intestinal fistulae have come under surgical control. Hospitalization for this nutritional support alone averages about $300 (£125) a day and can now be done at home for about one-tenth of that cost.

I have spent my life professionally in the care of what the world calls handicapped children. All of these had a physical defect to start with, some were habilitated to be indistinguishable from normal. Others were not pristine in form or function. Some had a mental handicap as well. They live and do well in families. They merely exist in institutions. I have seen many childless couples become a family when they took a handicapped child by adoption. Other traditional natural families have expanded by the same process. It all takes a tremendous investment in vision, time, effort, and money. There are tragedies and triumphs. But blessings frequently come with braces.

Notes

1. An artificial bladder made from a loop of small intestine.
2. The Raymond Pointcarré Hospital, Gausches.

Part 2
Potential in Disability

5. A MANY SPLENDOURED THING

Pat Seed

Life brings us many experiences. Some of them are pleasant, happy affairs and others are occasions we would rather erase from our memory. All experience has something to teach us. Unless we are prepared to learn, we cannot expect to grow in understanding, wisdom or compassion.

To have cancer and to have been given a medical prognosis of 6 months of life is not an experience one would seek. Having emerged from that traumatic situation and, so far, lived for four more years than was expected, what are my thoughts? Simply this: There is not one single thing a human being owns or possesses that is as important as *people* and human relationships.

1981 is the International Year of the Disabled. I suppose one could say that the whole human race is disabled in one way or another, in that none of us are perfect.

Indifference or prejudice may prevent understanding between people of various races and cultures, yet if each individual made a conscious effort to "love thy neighbour" no matter what the colour of his skin or his country of origin may be, the collective result could be profound.

From my own experiences, here are a few examples on the credit side and in contrast to those frequent reports of racial violence and animosity.

April 1976. . . I had returned to our local general hospital for the removal of deep tension sutures and for more tests, following a lapaerotomy operation. Cancer had been diagnosed and I was to be referred to the Christie Hospital and Holt Radium Institute, Manchester—Europe's largest cancer treatment centre. Cancer—the dreaded word which strikes fear into every human heart. What had I to hold on to?

I had the support of a loving family. As a Christian, I was clinging desperately to my trust in a God of Love who, I believe, has a reason for all things, even if at times we mere mortals are unable to comprehend. Sometimes, in retrospect, His purpose becomes known to us, yet I think the hardest words for any Christian to say—and mean—in times of stress or trouble are "Thy Will Be Done".

So there I was, sitting in a spotlessly clean bed and with my personal possessions stowed away in the bedside locker. My life as a wife, mother and journalist seemed to have come to a grinding halt. The future was an unknown quantity.

The ward was of the modern type, comprising several four bedded bays. Nurses moved quietly and efficiently, attending to patients and to their daily routine tasks. One other bed in my bay was occupied. In it was an elderly grey haired Asian lady. To establish contact and to take my mind off my own problems, I asked: "Are you in for an operation?"—she looked at me helplessly. After a few more attempts at conversation, it became apparent that she neither spoke nor understood English. I began to read a magazine, but from time to time, glanced at the patient in the next bed. Her hands plucked nervously at the sheets and occasional tears slid down her brown lined face. I was at a loss. Here was I, a journalist, a professional communicator, stymied by the language barrier. What could I do? That elderly lady could be someone's mother. How would I feel if my own mother was in a hospital bed in a strange land and unable to speak or understand the language.

"Oh God, how can I help her?" Was it a thought that came into my mind through sheer frustration, or was it a prayer? Whichever it was, it was immediately followed by a silent rebuke: "Don't be so inhibited—there's one language that is international!" Okay, so I might be rebuffed, but it was worth a try.

I got out of my bed and sat on hers. I smiled and in return a shy, yet apprehensive smile appeared on her face. Impulsively, I gathered her into my arms as though she were a child, drew her head onto my shoulder and stroked the grey hair. She cried. Then I held her so that I could look into her eyes. Putting my hand under her chin, I smiled again, winked at her and gave her a kiss. "Come on, you'll be alright— you'll see!" She didn't understand a word I said—but she got the message.

The international language—LOVE. In this instance, it had been simple and spontaneous and with no thought of being a "do-gooder".

At visiting time that evening, my husband arrived and a crowd of Asian people of various ages were gathered around the adjacent bed. Voluble conversation in a strange tongue ensued. When it was time for the visitors to leave, one of the younger men came to my bedside and said to me in English: "Thank you for your kindness to my Grandmother." To my astonishment, the entire family—nine of them, including two small children—shook hands with me as they left. As the old song has it, Love is a many splendoured thing.

For many months I did not recall this incident. My personal and then my public fight against cancer drove it from my mind. It came back to me when my Appeal Fund to buy a C.T. Scanner for the Christie Hospital was well established. I had been invited to a

Carribean Evening in aid of the Fund, organised by a local Ladies Circle. The music was provided by a West Indian Steel Band and as their melodious music filled the room, the President told me that the men had come straight from work on the late shift at a factory in a nearby town. Indicating one of the young men, she said: "His mother died of cancer a month ago."

I couldn't reply for the lump in my throat. That young man was using his talent to help others. We were fighting a common adversary—cancer. We were harnessed to the same yoke and the colour of our skins was of no consequence whatsoever.

Another incident which comes to mind is an evening when my husband and I visited two friends and their mentally handicapped son. When we arrived, they were watching television. On the screen a boxing match between a Nigerian and an Englishman was taking place. "Who do you think will win, Tim?" my husband asked the son of the house. "The one in the red shorts," was Tim's reply. That mentally handicapped boy, in his simplicity, displayed the wisdom of a Solomon.

I was reminded of the words of Malcolm Boyd:

I see white and black, Lord. I see white teeth in a black face.
I see black eyes in a white face. Help me to see persons, Jesus.
Not a black person, or a white person, a red person or a yellow
person, but human persons.

Cancer is a malignant random selector. It does not discriminate. The man on social security and the millionaire are equal candidates and the colour of one's skin is of no importance.

As I write this, a friend of mine is receiving treatment at the Christie for Leukaemia. A complete change of blood is needed, involving about 20 donors. Provided the blood group of each donor is compatible with that of the patient, it won't matter whether he or she was born in Tottenham, Thailand or Timbuctoo. My friend will be eternally grateful to all those human beings who help him in his dire need.

The Christie Hospital now has the most advanced and possibly the only purpose built C.T. Scanner department in the world. Since January 1980 it has helped well over 1,500 patients. Its installation was only made possible by *good* people of every race, creed and colour who saw fit to give—not just their money, but their time, talents and love.

Faith and hope founded a charity. It was love that transformed a seemingly impossible dream into a reality. Where love is, there God is also. For we ordinary human beings are His tools. His instruments—if we will let Him use us as *He* wills and not as we desire.

As St Teresa of Avila wrote in the sixteenth century:

Christ has no body now on earth but yours;
no hands but yours; no feet but yours.
Yours are the eyes through which is to look out Christ's compassion
to the world.
Yours are the feet with which he is to go about doing good.
Yours are the hands with which he is to bless men now

Yes—Love is a many splendoured thing. It's the most powerful force on earth and the international language. It doesn't cost money or need a high I.Q. to learn it. All each of us has to give is—ourself. The choice is yours.

6. MY HANDS AND I

John Steensma

There is such a tremendous multiplicity of disabilities in society today and conferences have made broad statements about the handicapped in the church, so I would like to make this a more personal presentation. I hope it will help you to understand where the disabled are coming from and where we, as a church, are in relationship to the disabled.

I lost my hands at the age of 17 in an electricity accident. It's difficult for you to imagine what it means to lose one or both hands. I'd like to help you by suggesting that you concentrate on your hands. Take a new look at them. "We are fearfully and wonderfully made,"[1] the Scriptures say. Hands are a miracle of engineering. Let me remind you of some of the beautiful aspects of hands.

First, the human arm and hand are tremendously flexible. When you pick something up, your hand automatically adapts to whatever size or shape it has. You can put your hand behind your back and you can put it out to your side. Another aspect of the human hand is its power. Each of you has an average power of grasp of from 100 to 130 pounds. The lifting power of the human hand and arm is amazing. If you use both hands, you can lift anywhere from 50 to 200 pounds from a dead weight. Weight-lifters can manage over 400 pounds. A boxer like Mohammed Ali can flatten your face with a 6 inch jab.

Next, sensation . . . I think this is one of God's most amazing gifts to human beings—the power to feel, to distinguish between hot and cold, soft and hard, smooth and rough. I often think of this in connection with the leprosy patients we have worked with. One effect of leprosy is the complete loss of feeling from the elbow down. Training these people to use their hands is like training someone to use artificial limbs. They have to be sensitive to whatever they are touching because their hands can become ulcerated very quickly.

The human hand has the ability to communicate too. Deaf people communicate with their hands; great orators have swayed audiences just with their gestures. The ability to communicate is important in our relationships with people—touching them, stroking their hair or their face, shaking hands with them. Hands identify us. In the United States, everyone is fingerprinted sometime during their life. It is a very distinct identification. So is the way we shake hands. We are very conscious of our hands. We dress them up—we spend thousands of dollars on soaps and creams and polishes and jewelry. We love our hands.

The Meaning of Disability caused by Accident or Illness

What happens if we lose them? One or both hands. We lose flexibility. You would not believe how many times you flex your wrist. If I want to get something out of my pocket, I have to think about it first. Your hand adjusts automatically to whatever you pick up, to its size and texture and temperature and weight. When I touch something with my eyes closed, I do not know what it is.

If I were to reach out and put my hook on the top of my neighbour's head as he sits beside me here, I am sure it would shake him up a bit if he did not know me. Because it would be the cold touch of steel. But because we know each other, I would be communicating and this would no longer be a steel hook touching him, it would be me, John Steensma. I love these hooks. I think they are beautiful because they do for me what your hands and fingers do for you. Without them I would have some real problems. It is all in how you look at it; it is all in the eye of the beholder.

Now, imagine that you are involved in a serious traffic accident and suffer a spinal cord injury which leaves you paralysed from the neck down. You will have to spend the rest of your life in a wheelchair. Or you have a massive stroke which results in the paralysis of one side of your body. There is some possibility of learning to walk again with a brace, but the arm does not regain its function. Speech is affected, either in the expression of words or in their reception, or both. The fact is, it is rare for people who have had a stroke to return to their employment.

The role of the comprehensive rehabilitation centre, such as the one with which my wife and I work, is to help restore these people to maximum function within the limits of their disability. Such a centre considers the whole person. At our rehabilitation centre, every medical discipline is represented. We have rehabilitation nurses, physical therapists, occupational therapists, social workers, psychologists, recreation therapists, work evaluators and vocational counsellors. We have a shop for manufacturing artificial limbs and braces. Our aim is the total rehabilitation of the individual, whatever his disability.

But then the person is discharged and goes back into the community where he came from. His real rehabilitation begins at the time of discharge. This is what the rehabilitation worker has been trying to do: to prepare the person for rejection and ostracism, to prepare him to cope with feeling incompetent and inadequate in the face of public attitudes and misunderstanding. To accept the possibility that he or she may have to find a whole new group of friends. Those in wheelchairs have to learn to accept their low posture which forces them to look up each time they talk to someone. They must get used to living in a society of insurmountable obstacles and architectural barriers and the difficulties of public transport. For others, there is the fear of embarrassment of a leaking catheter or an involuntary bowel movement. There are the feelings of inadequacy, diffidence and lack of confidence that his or her mate is not receiving sexual satisfaction. This last is a vital part of a disabled person's adjustment to disability and underscores the importance of counselling and instruction in new ways of sexual living.

Then there is the matter of finding employment that is adjusted to the person's particular disability. It means being denied a job for which you are otherwise qualified because of a physical disability. There are many agencies which serve the disabled, but they do not hire many of them. The United States is dealing with the problem very forcefully now, requiring employers to make reasonable accommodations and accessible premises for persons with disabilities. Being disabled also means facing up to the fact that some colleges and universities discriminate against you. It means living with the precarious hope that some day, medical science may be able to restore your physical functions. Finally, being disabled often means being treated as a non-person.

Attitudes to the Disabled

What does all this say to you and me? It is not an easy question to answer. We are talking about human relations, about individuals who are different—in age, in type of disability, in sex, ethnically; people with different sets of values.

To answer this question, let me suggest that we first know ourselves. What are our ambitions? Our goals? What are our tolerances and our prejudices? Can we stand to face people who are severely damaged or in crisis? Do we tend to become so emotionally involved that we hurt ourselves and hurt the other person? What do we really feel when we see a thoroughly disabled, spastic, drooling child?

May I also suggest that we do not stereotype people? Even today, when we speak of employing the mentally retarded, it is common to say, "Oh, they cannot do anything abstract . . ." This is just not true! The next suggestion I would have in encountering the disabled is—be yourself. Be just the way you are when you meet the un-disabled. For example, I have lectured to hundreds of special education students. I speak to them at the same personal gut level as I am doing now. Once one of those students asked me, "If I met you at the supermarket and was behind you at the cashier's, what should I say to you?" I told her, "The same thing you would say to anybody else." We are not freaks. I know I have a disability. Many people look upon it as abnormal. Some religious cults may consider a disability as a sign of punishment for past sins. But this simply should not be among Christians! I have lost my hands, but I am still the same person with the same drives, the same ambitions, the same desires, the same feelings as anybody else. This is true for all disabled people.

Be empathetic and yet objective. Bill Watty told us about the ailing parishioner whom he had visited and who recovered, got up and walked. I am sure his healing presence had something to do with it. He was empathetic and still, objective. He reached her. I would say this to all professionals, that if you establish a relationship with a patient which disturbs you so much that it keeps you awake at night, you should turn that person over to someone else because eventually, you are going to hurt them.

I have been reading a paper by a psychiatrist who has been working with severely damaged people for the past 30 years. He speaks of the professionals who serve these people and the damage they can inflict because they themselves have lost their empathy and become emotional and angry, feeling threatened.

We must be able to risk our emotions, especially as Christians. We have to take this risk because of the difference we could make to someone else. In the United States, for instance, we have lost the ability, or the art or the will, to touch people. We are afraid to, because touching has become so sexually-oriented. Yet this is part of risking your emotions—a touch can heal. So do not be afraid to touch people. Be observant, be consistently sensitive. Look at people! Be a listener. Do not be nice to somebody just because he or she is disabled. That is paternalistic and they can tell. I sometimes tell therapists to take 15 minutes out of their half-hour sessions with a patient and, instead of putting them through their exercises, just sit them down and listen. People in hospitals are lonely and dependent and often they are afraid. Listening to them is a way of healing. Be consistent—do not treat a person one way today and another way tomorrow. You may not feel the same way every day so it's hard to be consistent, but the disabled person is aware of this too. Be imaginative and be creative. There is always more than one way to solve a problem. Maybe your church can serve the function of being a place where disabled people can meet socially; maybe it can start some creative, imaginative programmes in your community. How can you get the disabled to come to church? In any community, 10% of the people are disabled in some way and many of them are in wheelchairs. What can you do about them? You can build a ramp or fix up a bathroom for them, but that is not creative. Anybody can do that.

After my accident, I was in hospital for almost 9 weeks. There was never a doubt in my mind that when I returned home, I was still going to be John Steensma—a son, a brother. My mother told me, "John, you're home now. I know you need help, but you are going to be independent. We are not going to coddle you, but we'll love you."

I knew my neighbours and my friends would accept me. Even before I had my prothesis, one of them came and said, "John, how about going on a double date tonight? I'll drive." I did not want to go, but I did. That was back in the days of chivalry too, when men still opened doors for ladies and held their coats. I was ahead of my time.

Helen Keller once said: "The person who is severely impaired, never knows his hidden sources of strength until he or she is treated like a normal human being and encouraged to shape his or her own life." Here is another quotation I would like to share with you: "Even the most severely disabled people retain an indefatigable conviction that they are still human in all that is ultimately necessary."

There will always be problems wherever there are human wills and emotions, different personalities and varying degrees of emotional and spiritual desires. How we work out the differences is what counts.

We cannot and should not even attempt to predetermine the potential of any individual. For the severely disabled, the mere fact of living and being dependent is difficult. However, we should be able to provide the sympathetic understanding which recognises this dependence while at the same time, gently guiding him or her back to independence. This requires tact, sympathy, sensitivity, wisdom and the imagination to recognise the person's potential which he or she may not even know. We must see this unlimited potential. This is not idealism. It is reality.

Note

1. Ps 139 vs 14.

7. THE SITUATION IN DEVELOPING COUNTRIES

*Stuart Kingma**

I

Definitions

The United Nations' Organisations have designated 1981 as the International Year of Disabled Persons. Individuals and organisations around the world are mobilizing to respond to this initiative on behalf of those 500 million members of the human family who, every day, carry with them some form of impairment or disability. The changes we are all looking for are fundamental, pervasive and far-reaching. The accomplishment of these changes will require a solid commitment on the part of everyone. All of us need to begin by understanding much more clearly what the nature of physical and mental impairment really is, what is the full range of effects these impairments have upon the lives of those who have disabilities, and what is needed to permit disabled persons to participate fully in their own lives and within family and society.

All of this needs to begin with an educational process. Architectural change is another part of the process, to permit people with disabilities to have free access to buildings and services. The prevention and treatment of impairment require much greater emphasis within all of our programmes, and particularly those related to the healing professions. Rehabilitation is another critical activity which will demand a new and creative approach if its services are to be made available to all of those who could benefit from it.

It may be helpful to begin with a few definitions. The following formulation is taken from a recent document of the World Health Organisation (WHO) *International Classification of Impairments, Disabilities and Handicaps* (1980):

Impairment: In the context of health experience, an impairment is any loss or abnormality of psychological, physiological or anatomical structure or function. An impairment may be temporary or permanent, and it includes the existence or occurrence of an anomaly, defect or loss in a limb, organ, tissue or other structure of the body, or a defect in a functional system or mechanism of the body, including the systems of mental function. An impairment may cause functional limitations which are the partial or total inability to perform those activities

---

*   This paper is adapted from an article taken from *Contact* the bi-monthly bulletin of the Christian Medical Commission of the World Council of Churches.

usually carried out by the organ or systems affected. In principle, impairments represent disturbances at the organ or system level.

Disability: In the context of health experience, a disability is any restriction or lack (resulting from an impairment) of ability to perform an activity in the manner or within the range considered normal for a human being. This is concerned with compound or integrated activities expected of the person or of the body as a whole, such as are represented by tasks, skills and behaviours. Disabilities thus represent disturbances at the level of the person. In this connection, it is preferable to say that someone has a disability, a statement which preserves neutrality and implies that person's potential still being possible. To say that someone is disabled risks describing the individual with a more pervasive concept and stigma.

Handicap: In the context of health experience, a handicap is a disadvantage for a given individual, resulting from an impairment or disability, that limits or prevents the fulfilment of a role that is normal (depending on age, sex, and social and cultural factors) for that individual. A handicap is thus a social phenomenon, representing the social and environmental consequences for the individual, stemming from the presence of impairments and disabilities. The ideas and concepts just described can be linked in the following manner:

DISEASE or			
DISORDER______	IMPAIRMENT___	DISABILITY_____	HANDICAP
(intrinsic	(exteriorized)	(objectified)	(socialised)
situation)			

Many factors play important roles in the origin of an impairment and its resulting functional limitation and disability. These causative factors include specific medical causes related to the individual, environmental factors, attitudes and other sociocultural determinants and social demands. Table 1 (p.46) is an estimate provided by the WHO of the causes of disability and the estimated number of disabled people, by cause, in the world.

Prevention and Rehabilitation

Interventions aimed at reducing the occurrence of disability or at diminishing its impact fall into two main categories which can be termed "disability prevention" and "rehabilitation". The prevention of disability includes a variety of activities including those which act upon the individual directly (treatment, counselling, prosthetics, medical care, training, etc.) those which act upon the individual's

immediate surroundings (family, community, employer attitudes and
behaviour towards the individual etc.) and those with the broad aim
of reducing risks occurring in society as a whole.

Table 1

CAUSES OF DISABILITY AND ESTIMATED NUMBER OF DISABLED PEOPLE IN THE WORLD[1]

Medical Cause	Estimated disabled people (world population 4000 million)	
	Millions	%
Congenital disturbances:		
Mental retardation[2]	40	7.7
Somatic hereditary defects	40	7.7
Non-genetic disorders	20	3.9
Communicable diseases:		
Poliomyelitis	1.5	0.3
Trachoma	10	1.9
Leprosy	3.5	0.7
Onchocerciasis	1	0.2
Other communicable diseases	40	7.7
Non-communicable		
Somatic disease	100	19.3
Functional psychiatric disturbance	40	7.7
Chronic alcoholism and drug abuse	40	7.7
Trauma/injury:[3]		
Traffic accidents	30	5.8
Occupational accidents	15	2.9
Home accidents	30	5.8
Other	3	0.6
Malnutrition	100	19.3
Other	2	0.4
TOTAL	516	100.0
Correction for possible double accounting (-25%)	-129	
TOTAL	387	

Rehabilitation is usually defined as the third phase in medicine (prevention being the first and curative care the second), and this term is used to define such interventions as in general aimed at providing treatment and services to patients who are already disabled or at great risk of disablement because of an existing functional limitation. It is "the combined and coordinated use of medical, social, educational and vocational measures for training or retraining the individual to the highest possible level of functional ability".

II

Current Situation

An analysis of the current situation allows us to make certain statements about future trends in the magnitude and characteristics of the disability problem. Again, I draw heavily on WHO for this analysis.

Efforts to control communicable diseases are a continuing commitment of governments and non-governmental agencies, and if there is a future decrease in morbidity from these diseases, certain types of disabilities will be reduced. On the other hand, greater survival through improved medical care for disabling illnesses may contribute to an increase in certain types of disability.

The world food situation is a matter of continuing concern, and present trends show a steady increase in the problem of malnutrition. This will lead to an increase in the number of persons disabled as a result of the immediate and long-term effects of under-nutrition.

The changing age composition in the world and extending life expectancy in many countries will certainly contribute to changes in the characteristics of the disability problem.

Increased urbanization and industrialisation also contribute to increasing disability problems. The factors here are multiple and complex, but certainly include road and industrial accidents as well as the psychological pressures of urbanization.

Problems Particular to Developing Countries

The problem faced by developing countries is particularly great. This is true not only because the number of people with significant disabilities is undoubtedly larger in these countries compared to the total population, but also because of the limited resources which these countries have at their disposal to respond to the needs of disabled persons.

47

A brief example will serve to illustrate this point. Botswana is a country of relatively low population in southern Africa and it is among the countries referred to by the United Nations as one of the least developed countries. The current population is estimated to be around 700,000. A study was recently made of the needs of disabled people in Botswana for the purposes of planning for an expanded service of rehabilitation in the country.[4] This study began with the basic assumption that, within any population, 10% of the people have medical, social and economic problems related to disability. At least one in ten of these, or some 7,000 people, would be in immediate need and can benefit from rehabilitation services. At that time, the country had very little organised rehabilitation actually functioning. Institutions run by non-governmental organisations had a combined capacity of about 60 persons and could admit about 20 new people with disabilities per year. There was a clear need to further extend services to reach more of the population in need.

Village-based Treatment

The first option open to the planners would be to provide more specialised rehabilitation institutions of the type already established, institutions which would be considered the conventional response. For this option, capital costs would obviously be very high, and the need for professionals to run these services would demand between 700 and 1,000 highly trained people. However, in addition to these facts, it was conservatively estimated that the running costs for this conventional response, if the needs of these 7,000 people would be met, would amount to twice the total annual budget for the Ministry of Health.

Obviously, some new and creative thinking was needed for Botswana as it is needed for other countries as well. One option suggested by this study is that of community-based rehabilitation; this required no institutions except for a few referral stations which would be developed later in response to community needs. The total professional staff required is less than 20, and the annual running costs would be equivalent to about 2% of the national health budget. In this approach, basic rehabilitation would be carried out in the community itself and usually within the home of the disabled person. This would consist of simple therapy, the provision of simple technical aids made locally, teaching in order to restore the capacity to participate in the activities of daily living, the provision of work situations appropriate to the specific disability and other social measures.

This effort has taken into consideration the fact that the effectiveness of conventional institutions is seriously questioned now because they so often run counter to the objective of keeping disabled people within the mainstream of life. The rehabilitation itself is entrusted to primary health care workers and other community members including family members. Government and non-governmental organisations are all drawn into the total effort. This is the kind of creative thinking and planning which will be demanded of all of us during this year and for the years to come.

Perhaps one other illustration will serve to reinforce this point. Southern Asia is known to carry a heavy burden of eye problems and has a high incidence of blindness. It is estimated that of the 15 million blind people in the world, 5.8 million are in India alone. About 30% of these blind people are believed to lose their eyesight from *preventable childhood illnesses*. Another very large percentage are from other diseases which are either preventable or can be treated at an early enough stage to prevent the loss of eyesight. In the South India State of Kerala, a project has been under way for some $2\frac{1}{2}$ years under the joint auspices of the Christoffel-Blindenmission of the Federal Republic of Germany and the MGDM Hospital in Kangazha. This *Preservation of Eyesight Project*[5] has concentrated on the prevention of blindness through measures taken at the village level, using specifically trained village health workers. The training programme utilized volunteers selected by their own communities, and the training lasted 8 weeks. In addition to a supervisory level of worker, a referral system was utilized for support from the base hospital. The activities at the village concentrated on the prevention of vitamin A deficiency, nutritional programmes to prevent protein-calorie malnutrition, the prevention of childhood diseases through immunisation, the early detection and treatment of eye diseases, screening for the detection of cataract, glaucoma, diabetes and hypertension, a school programme to screen the vision and treat refracted errors in children, and the rehabilitation of blind people through vocational training. The results have shown a remarkable reduction in many of the most serious eye threatening problems and a new awareness of both the value of prevention and the possibilities for severely disabled people to re-enter the mainstream of life through training.

A similar project in the neighbouring Indian State of Tamil Nadu[6] also makes use of the village-level field worker for the purposes of screening for eye problems, training blind people in the activities of daily living, vocational training and follow-up. An extensive experience has been developed in this project in the training of these disabled people in many specific activities to enable them to become fully independent in and around their own villages.

The World Health Organization itself is undertaking a programme of prevention in the Himalayan State of Nepal where, among its 12 million people, a quarter of a million are known to be blind. Ninety per cent of the blindness identified in a survey carried out two years ago was found to be either preventable or curable. The aim of this programme is to focus on the preventive efforts that can be carried out within the communities to eliminate the huge burden of avoidable blindness in that country. The bulk of the work will be carried out by village health workers, and a health education campaign has been launched for the population in five priority areas. Drugs and basic instruments will be made available to all district and health post centres and an ophthalmic eye unit will begin to function in the very near future.

Handicapped Children

Thanks to a study of the situation of handicapped children being carried out by Rehabilitation International with assistance from the United Nations Children's Fund—UNICEF—we have in recent months had the opportunity of observing the lives of children with disabilities in villages and slums in Bangladesh and Mexico, the Philippines and Jamaica, Kenya and India and Saudi Arabia and Brazil. These experiences have more than verified our estimates as to the prevalence of impairment, they have demonstrated the almost universal absence of relevant services for these people, and they have forced us again to feel and taste and smell the degradation of human life which is its only promise for those millions of people.

Thanks to these and other observations of the situation in the developing areas, I am able to offer some generalizations that I am certain are valid for the great majority of the people living in such areas.

Disability and Poverty

The first has to do with the dreadful implications of the combination of disability and poverty. Either one may cause the other, and their presence in combination has a tremendous capacity to destroy the lives of people with impairments and to impose on families burdens that are too crushing to bear.

We have not come to grips with the interactions between these two forces—the frequency with which untreated impairment starts or accelerates the collapse of a family's already fragile economic base, the degree to which social and economic deprivation are fundamental causes of impairment, and of the escalation of impairment into permanent disability. We do not yet think of services to prevent impairment and to rehabilitate disabled persons as being basic components of economic and social development because we have not yet faced the evidence to be found out there in the villages and barrios and favelas that they are.

"Relief" Does Not Aid Disabilities

Second, we are finding that, when programmes to assist in the development of the community reach it, the benefits go last and least to those families that are burdened with both poverty and disability. This is a consequence of many factors within the family, the society and the fragility of human compassion, but in the end it is usually because the family with a disabled member has been to some degree rejected from the mainstream of community life and resources—and there is nothing in the development plan to counteract that social reality.

Within the family, it is too often the child with the impairment who is denied the chance for better food, for education, for medical care, for social and intellectual stimulation, even when these benefits do become available to his or her sisters and brothers.

Lack of Information

Third, and directly connected with everything I am saying, there is an abysmal lack of accurate information about disability, its causes and consequences, and about what we can do about these things; and an equally appalling wealth of misinformation, prejudice, superstition and fear. This is a major factor in the family's inadequate reaction to the problem when it arises; it is a fundamental reason for the community's ostracising individuals and families that are affected with disability; it exists in the institutions that might be helping, but aren't—the health centre, the school, the religious grouping; it permeates all echelons of government from the village chief to the ministers of health, education, welfare, labour, community development, planning and whatever else may exist; and it is endemic in the representatives of international and other organisations who are advising on the procedures and priorities of development, and administering international assistance. This absence of information and understanding, and the manner in which it reinforces the traditional distorted concepts of disability which flourish throughout the world, does much to conceal the real magnitude of the problem and to confuse everyone's thinking about the solutions.

Disability is Socially Unacceptable

Fourth, these factors combine to produce attitudes and patterns of individual and social behaviour that are themselves important causes of disability and of handicapped lives in the developing countries—just as they are in Washington, D.C. As I have said, children with even minor impairments are often stigmatized as crippled or blind or deaf or retarded and shut off from the very support and stimulation that would enable them to develop and function in society. Adults with certain categories of disability, varying with traditions and culture, are denied participation in the basic forms of social life—the productive activities of the community, its institutions of government, marriage and parenthood—more because of the stigma attached to disability than because it practically limits the capacity for action.

These social forces are not unique to the developing areas; they are well-known in every part of the world. In general, however, people living in the least developed areas function in what Edward Hall has termed a "high context" social situation. The individual's role in the community is much more rigidly defined by the circumstances of the family and its traditional relationships, and his or her self-image and confidence are derived from the capacity to fulfil that role in the social context in which it has been evolved. Thus when, because of the functional limitations associated with an impairment or because of the stigmatization of the disabled person, he or she is not permitted to grow into and fulfil the traditional role, the individual is very likely to become a non-person, an outcast without value to self, to the family or to the community. The importance of this factor must not be overlooked when planning interventions into the situation—but it usually is.

Unsuitable Rehabilitation Reaches Very Few Handicapped

Fifth, at least 90% and probably more of whatever rehabilitation services exist in the developing areas have been designed and activated on the basis of models found in the industrialised West, and have been assisted and staffed by people trained in those models. This international cooperation and assistance has taken place almost entirely in the past 30 years. It has produced some islands of excellence—centres, schools and programmes that are performing as well as the models from which they have been derived—and workers of great dedication and skill.

Two crucial problems remain. First, the totality of the existing services reach at best a few thousand people in the areas where we estimate there are at least 300 million with disabilities and an additional two million each year. And second, we may question whether the concepts of rehabilitation services which have evolved in the industrialised West are necessarily appropriate for areas with quite different economic and social situations.

I believe that, in order to help our friends in the developing areas to design and activate services that will have some hope of reaching a more significant proportion of their disabled people, and to do it in a way that will improve the lives of the people concerned according to their values, not ours, we need to do some new thinking.

It may be useful first to review some of the main characteristics of the models we have been exporting. If they have been faulty, I do not think we must necessarily have great pangs of guilt. After all, during the past 30 years, we ourselves have been learning what disability and rehabilitation are all about; and today, we are still struggling to overcome traditions and prejudices that continue to limit the effectiveness of our services and to offend the rights of people with disabilities. We have been exporting what we thought was best, and we are just beginning to understand how much the concepts we have been using have concealed from us, as well as from the people in developing areas, the greater potentials for more useful action that exist.

The "Western" Model

The rehabilitation model, which has dominated the scene both in the industrialised West and in our international assistance activity has three working parts; fancy buildings, elaborate equipment and highly specialised professional personnel. We have evolved standards for each of these components in the most sophisticated setting with unlimited research and development funds, and have cloaked these standards in an aura so sacred that our friends in the developing world are led to believe that anything different is unacceptable, and that what is being done in Zurich or Copenhagen or Houston is, by divine mandate, appropriate for Kaduna, Semarang and Caruaru.

Professional Remote Services

Our emphasis has been on services that the professional will give to the disabled person and, to a lesser extent, to the family. We have said, "Bring your disabled person to our "magic house," with our charmed equipment and our inspired specialists, and we will change him or her and send him or her back to you, less disabled and better able to cope in your community." But we have also had to say, depending on the circumstances, "We can take only those of you who can pay our charges, or who are within the neighbourhood of the magic house, or who can come back three times a week for six months, or who have transportation, or who are willing to accept our definition of your future."

It has been our practice, and the burden of the example we export, to lift both the problem and the person with the problem out of the social context in which they exist and to attempt to find a solution in a new context of our making. We have only slowly learned that a person with a disability is also a person with a lot of other things: with a family, with traditions, with customs, with tastes and appetites, with fears and apprehensions, with pride and ambitions, and with a culture through which these elements are integrated. Whether we have brought people from South America to New York for rehabilitation or whether we have advised the construction of large and comprehensive centres in the capital cities of South America, the foundation of the thinking we have exported has been to remove the individual from everything in his or her life except the impairment and to concentrate on that. We have, to all practical purposes, ignored the rich array of support that is ready to be activated in the community, in the family, and in the individual with the impairment.

My sixth and seventh points are ideas that apply to all international aid for development, and are directly relevant to our concerns:

The sixth is the principle of social magnetism. It says that, by and large, when we venture into the developing world, we find our greatest empathy with the people there who can speak our language, who share some of our ideas about how society should be organised and with whom we feel comfortable. People who meet these criteria are of course usually people who, for one reason or another, have had a Western education and acculturation, who understand the conceptual basis on which our human assistance programmes are based, and who aspire for a similar, abeit inappropriate, set of services in their countries. Please understand me, some of my dearest friends in the world are in the category I have just described, and I fully understand the roles they have played in motivating developing activity; but the hard reality is that they do not always comprehend the real dimensions of the disability problem as it affects all the people of their countries, and their reinforcement of our parochial concepts does not necessarily mean that they are relevant. Our most important challenge is to understand what disability means to the person and the family in the village of Bangladesh, in the urban slum of Brazil—and the people with whom we normally associate in those countries cannot usually give us the answer.

The seventh point is also applicable to all development activity. It concerns the collapse of the "trickle-down" theory. We have assumed that, by stimulating and assisting the establishment of showplace institutions in capital cities, we would start a trickling-down process that would eventually diffuse appropriate levels of service to the smaller communities. When we have talked about national programmes, we have referred to networks of showplace centres which would trickle down. It hasn't happened, and we should now know that it won't happen unless there is a very hard-headed plan, based on the realities of both resources and culture, to activate it.

III

Recommended Improvements

What can we do to get a better result from the resources we expect to put into the improvement of the life of disabled persons in areas in the earlier stages of development? Let me suggest some principles that I think should be considered.

Prevention

I haven't said much about prevention, but this should not imply that I do not think it important. It is completely obvious that we will never effectively reduce the problem of disability until we do something intelligent about reducing the incidence of impairment. Look at the major causes—malnutrition, birth defects, diseases and accidents—and at the multifaceted action necessary to reduce their tragic consequences. Obviously a vast task, but one that we cannot put aside if we want to reduce the problem of disability.

We need not go into all the details which are involved in current international discussions as to the definitions of impairment, disability and handicap but thinking about them does clarify our ideas about prevention and about the fact that it can be applied at every level.

We can prevent the impairment by preventing the malnutrition, the birth defect, the disease or the accident; if it happens, we can prevent the permanent disability by effective care and treatment; and we can prevent so many of the real social consequences, the handicap, by intelligent social action and public education programmes. If you are shopping for an activitiy that will be efficient in reducing the incidence of disability in the developing areas, look at one of the many aspects of prevention.

We have made a major mistake in separating prevention and rehabilitation. The human experience is a progressive development which starts before conception, when the characteristics of the mating partners may or may not produce impairment,[7] and terminates at death which too often is the culmination of a progressive reduction of capacities, a process which in other contexts we call disability. Whether it will be called a disability depends on the culture more than on the incapacity.

Our programmes and the programmes we have urged upon the developing countries, are not based on these realities. They are based on the idea that an impairment is a special event, and that it requires that the recipient be immediately removed from the normal stream of development and performance, and introduced to the blessings of our buildings, equipment and professional personnel.

55

Prevention, Rehabilitation and Social Action

I would like to suggest that we try to establish and to discuss with our friends in the developing countries, an understanding that the whole process is a continuum of prevention, rehabilitation and social action. These are not separate crusades, they are interlocking and interacting components of a system whose only purpose is to support the optimum development of each individual's capacity and personality. Our planning, and the planning we discuss with the developing countries, should be an extension of that concept.

Disability is a Cause of Under-Development

A very important function of our international assistance activity is what we might call advocacy, the model we present and the kind of policies we advocate. I said earlier that ignorance of the problem of disability, of its consequences and of its solutions is a characteristic of most of our colleagues who are advising governments about their development plans. This is tragically true despite certain heart-warming but rare exceptions. And so I would say that a high priority must be given to convincing everyone who deals in policy about these things that disability is an important cause and consequence of under-development, and that dealing with it must be a priority item in any intelligent development plan. Not the least important function at this level is that of refining the concepts we have been discussing and of giving them a practical relevance to the economic and social possibilities of the developing countries.

Existing Personnel Ready to Help

A next concern is with what we grandiosely call the infrastructure. Because of our involvement with, what are thought of locally, as the "magic house, the charmed equipment and the inspired specialists", we have generally overlooked the potential contribution of the people and institutions which, having more general objectives, nevertheless can and should be helping us. During the UNICEF-assisted study I mentioned earlier, Rehabilitation International has talked with a great many village health workers, teachers, social security agents, political and religious leaders, community development motivators and others who should be ready to assist in this area. The pervasive lack of information I mentioned earlier applies, and also there is an absence of understanding and spirit and motivation that must be corrected if we are to change the situation.

Improving Understanding and Motivation

It is probable that one of the most important objectives of any international assistance activity to the developing areas should be to improve the understanding and the motivation of people in the related services—health, education, vocational and welfare—towards their clients with disabilities.

The most important asset for any programme for disability prevention and rehabilitation is the family, and in most developing areas the ties and functions of the family are strong components of the social context of the individual. We should give a much higher priority to activities that will overcome the superstitions and fears of the members of the families of disabled persons, instruct them in procedures they can follow to prevent disability or assist the rehabilitation process, and acquaint them with the sources of help that may be or become available. Successful work at this level, by remaining within the existing social framework of the individual's life, can do much to maintain normal human development and performance whether or not the impairment can be eliminated or reduced.

The "General Rehabilitation" Worker

For many years we have talked about the potential utility of a "general rehabilitation worker" who would be trained to function at the community level and to perform some of the activities needed there. Conceptions have varied with circumstances, but generally have included such functions as early identification of the signs of impairment and other case finding, liaison with community or nearby sources that might be drawn upon, supervising and monitoring home treatment, assisting in the fabrication or procurement of simple technical aids, and other similar tasks. Experiments have also taken place to add such primary functions to the mission of community development activators, health promoters and others already working at the community level.

To my knowledge, we have not yet found a fully workable solution in any setting, bearing in mind that the definition of the responsibilities of this general worker will no doubt be different in different parts of the world. There are of course individuals whose motivations, personalities and energies enable them to give the kinds of help I have mentioned, but I know of no place where such general rehabilitation workers are trained and placed in the field on a systematic basis. I believe that it is an idea which merits further study and testing through demonstration projects that could well be supported by international assistance.

National Programmes for Prevention and Rehabilitation

It is obvious that there must be, whenever the resources permit, a chain of services which will provide the specialised care and treatment that will be required by some people and will be referral sources for those working in the field. It certainly should be a function of international assistance to train people and to provide equipment for such services, but this development should always be seen as a part of an overall national programme for disability prevention and rehabilitation, and be linked to the referral chain down to the village where most of the problems exist.

More Appropriate Information

All of the objectives I have cited require a much more adequate flow of appropriate kinds and levels of information. From the approaches needed to improve the orientation of international planners and ministers of health to the most simple instructions prepared to assist an illiterate mother in dealing with an impaired child, from general guidance for village health workers to suggestions for teachers who have exceptional pupils, and particularly for people with disabilities, very little of the printed and audiovisual material we have is appropriate or effective. Experience has been gained in achieving these kinds of communications in other fields, and must be combined with our own experience of the problems we are discussing so that we can produce, or stimulate and support the production of materials in the languages or imagery needed and at the levels of the target audiences.

I am aware that I have both over-simplified and over-generalised the situation, and that there are examples of progress supported by international assistance that are more positive than I have described. I will continue, however, to defend the thesis that the situations I have described are those in which the great majority of disabled people in the developing world (and indeed in most industrialised societies) are living, and that the characteristics I have ascribed to most of our efforts to assist them are accurate—the evidence is out there to prove it.

SUMMARY

I   International definitions of IMPAIRMENT, DISABILITY and HANDICAP. Table 1. p.46 gives an estimate provided by the WHO of the causes of disability and the estimated number of disabled people, by cause, in the world.

Disability can be reduced by two categories of intervention: disability prevention and rehabilitation. Both can affect either individuals in their immediate surroundings or can be aimed to reduce risks occurring in the society as a whole.

II   The second section is an analysis of the current situation particularly in developing countries, examples are taken from Botswana and India.

Developing countries tend to have a large proportion of disabled people in their populations but smaller resources. Consequently, it is argued, new thinking by National governments and countries giving aid is required. It is necessary that countries willing to give material or financial help should understand what disability means in the disabled person's home surroundings.

On the basis of observations made largely by UNICEF, the authors can point to the main effects of impairment and handicap.

Poverty combined with handicap can destroy a family. What begins as a comparatively minor handicap can develop into impairment and permanent disability through lack of access to any source of help.

It is often a child with an impairment who is not given access to better food or free services. There is very little information about disability generally available in developing countries.

If an impairment means that an individual in an under-developed country is unable to play the role in society expected of them they are inevitably judged socially inferior.

Aid-giving countries have tended to take handicapped people out of their own home surroundings to a "western style" institution. By so doing and thereby overlooking those at local level who could be trained to help, far fewer handicapped people can be rehabilitated and less impairment prevented.

It has been recognised by many people involved in aid to developing countries that help will not automatically spread from well-equipped centres to poor rural areas without a great deal of pressure.

III   The third section suggests some action which might improve the situation.

Prevention in any one of many ways is the most obvious way to improve the occurrence of impairments leading to permanent handicap.

Prevention, rehabilitation and social action at a local level are inter-related.

It is important to demonstrate to those who plan aid programmes to what a large extent disability is an important cause and consequence of under-development.

More attention should be paid to the availability of locally trained personnel such as village health workers, teachers, social security agents, political and religious leaders, community development motivators and others who would be ready to assist in this area.

In turn, more education should be directed to overcoming the fears and superstitions of the handicapped person's immediate family.

The idea of the "General Rehabilitation Worker" whose function would vary in different circumstances, should be encouraged by further testing and international support.

Help in prevention and rehabilitation with the necessary personnel and local services should be part of an overall National programme, not an isolated effort.

Much more relevant, accurate and appropriate information could be collected and disseminated to the right authorities. This would go some way to ensure that prevention and rehabilitation connected with disablement would receive appropriate international support.

Notes

1. Table 1 is taken from "Disability Prevention and Rehabilitation" *Reports on Technical Matters* 29th World Health Assembly Document A29/INF.Doc.1 WHO.
2. Not all of these are congenital cases.
3. Details of the further sub-classification *non-accidental and accidental injury in children* are also available from the appropriate National Statistics Departments.
4. Helander, E. *Personal Communication.*
5. Joseph, Y.V., *Preservation of Eyesight Project* and *Experiment in Prevention of Blindness at Community Level* (Unpublished manuscript, August, 1980).
6. Jahle, R., "Rehabilitation of Blind Persons in Rural India" *Journal of Visual Impairment and Blindness*, June 1977.
7. For the international definition see p.44 of this paper.

Part 3
Dignity in Dying

8. A CHRISTIAN VIEW OF HEALING

Dr. G. Scorer M.L. F.R.C.S.

The public life of Jesus as told in the Four Gospels shows many examples of Jesus' Healing Ministry. We are also informed of the vast numbers of people living in Israel at the time who came to Jesus for healing. "The whole town gathered at the door."[1] And later, "Jesus could no longer enter a town openly but stayed outside in lonely places. Yet the people still came to Him from everywhere".[2]

To see the public ministry of Jesus of Nazareth merely as an example for doctors to follow is to look at one facet only of a precious diamond. Jesus made it quite clear that his healing work was only part of something much greater. His healing of the body represented a struggle for the human soul. Healing of sickness was a foretaste of his conquest of death through his crucifixion and resurrection from the dead. The whole is so much more important than a single part.

If we look more closely at other Christian dimensions of healing we shall find them also in the person and redeeming work of Christ. We will briefly mention some important aspects.

Service

The story of the Good Samaritan has been absorbed into medical thinking over countless centuries and is still our brightest inspiration. Its penetrating insights into human nature are easily overlooked. My "neighbour" whom I serve cannot be designated merely by bed, or list, or appointment, or locality. He is any man or woman in need, whom I happen to meet as I go about my routine activities. Love does not discriminate between persons. Service can never be casual or perfunctory, or a chore. The Samaritan followed through his first aid by foreseeing the needs for the future and making provision for them in the donkey, the inn, the twopence and a return visit.

Organisations to help the sick and the disabled, the infant and the aged have multiplied in the last few decades. However, the most efficient and comprehensive organisations are only a scaffolding within which caring human hearts can build. If love of others is lacking, criticism and disillusion will take its place.

The Christian dimension in Medicine is not to be found in the structure or organisation of health services but in the character of the doctor himself and the manner in which he practises. In Western Medicine, over the past few centuries, we have known the leadership of many strong men and women who have laid firm foundations. But foundations can crumble. They need to be kept constantly in good repair. The heart of medical practice is, and always will be, the encounter between the doctor and his patient who needs help.

Human Life

What impressed many and so irritated the Religious Leaders during Jesus' life on earth was the way Jesus identified with the least popular among the people, the outcasts of polite society (though these were obviously not kept in institutions at that time). He touched the untouchable. The timid woman, the vociferous foreigner, the notorious whore, the soldier of the occupying power and the despised Samaritan, all came to Him for help. He brought life to the dead and restored full activity to the disabled. He loved life.

Such concern for human life is rooted in Old Testament teaching where, from conception to its physical dissolution, all life is regarded as being under God's personal protection. He is as much concerned with the foetus in the womb and the elderly without all their faculties as with the leaders of nations or the young in their prime. The sanctity of human life is a Christian concept from which we derive a principle which should at all times be the foundation of medical practice. It is surely a principle of which we as a profession should be proud and we should never let it go.

If we take enough time to find out, every life however apparently diminished and distorted is the life of an individual person. The Christian attitude to life enriches society, whether it inspires a Thomas Barnado receiving every destitute child in London's East End, Mother Teresa caring for unwanted babies in Calcutta, lone missionaries serving the leprosy rejects of undeveloped nations or Cicely Saunders putting hope and serenity back into the lives of those dying from cancer. At the present time it is largely Christians who try to prevent the taking of life through abortion and "mercy killing".

Human Suffering and Death

If the Christian is one who loves life and is committed to protecting it, he is at the same time, someone who has come to terms with suffering and death. Though death is inevitable for everyone, it never need be without hope. Suffering is an experience which can be very bitter and long lasting to a few. Whether it is due to the kind of world we live in, with its genetic disorders, diseases, injuries and other afflictions or whether it is part of "man's inhumanity to man", it has to be faced and if possible transformed. Dean Inge pointed out[3] that Christ as God and man threw new light on suffering and death through his crucifixion and apparent rejection by the Father. In consequence there is no way Christians can avoid the problem or recommend a "quick way out". Doctors have to face the problem of suffering and death as Christians, as well as doctors trained for the relief of suffering.

If the Christian is one who loves life and will not retreat from the problem of suffering he is, at the same time, someone who has come to terms with death. Death is not a catastrophe, or an ignominious and unmentionable experience, or an admission of inevitable medical failure. It is a door through which everyone must go. Since a doctor will almost inevitably be involved with terminal illness he is especially involved with dying. The doctor, if he is to serve his patient well, needs to be a particular kind of person.

Notes

1. Mark I:33
2. Mark I:45
3. *Speculum Animae* by W. R. Inge

9. IS "MERCY KILLING" NECESSARY?

Dr. Thomas West

The interface between expertise and expediency has become a major area of conflict in our time. The following chapter is taken from a debate originally printed in the *Journal of the Royal Society of Medicine*, (Vol 72, June 1979) and used with their permission.

St. Christopher's Hospice was created by Dame Cicely Saunders as a focal point of care and as a springboard for the "Hospice Movement" which is world wide and firmly based on good medicine.

The professions concerned with "care" must present their case to the profession concerned with "law" and trust that the experts, having distinguished between expediency and true expertise, will translate into sound law the evidence that is put before them. The concept of "mercy killing" acquiesces in the wrong remedy for an ill remediable by better means. In 14 years St. Christopher's has cared for over 7,000 patients, a great number of whom have been referred for the control of uncontrolled pain, and not of physical pain alone. Criteria for admission to the Hospice include unresolved mental, social and spiritual pain as well.

Case History

I admitted Mrs. O to St. Christopher's from a local hospital on 19th May 1977. She had an inoperable carcinoma of the pancreas with secondary deposits in the liver. She was in severe pain. The medical student with me was appalled at her suffering.

On the application form was written, "She does not know she has carcinoma." On questioning she said to me, "When you have pain for a year you start to think!" Of course she knew. By listening to her story, (she had had a very sad marriage) and observing her carefully, a correct assessment was made of the physical and the mental components of her pain and the correct drugs were prescribed. Within a few days she admitted that the pain was under control for the first time for a year.

She did not remain completely pain-free. But each Monday she had her hair washed and set, each Thursday she visited our weekly bar, and each Sunday she came to chapel. The ward staff soon learned that with meticulous attention to her drugs, and with even more attention to herself, when pain did break through, it could almost always be alleviated.

She was with us just under 3 months. Her last few days were peaceful and pain-free and she died surrounded by three faithful friends, the ward sister and a nurse. A few days later one of her friends wrote: "When I visited her in a previous hospital she was like a demented animal consumed with pain . . . I was very frightened, not knowing how to cope . . . I saw her at St. Christopher's restored to the dignity of a calm rational human being . . . from then on I was able to remain with her for hours, instead of minutes . . . discussing things dear to her heart . . . By so doing I, too, have gained in spiritual strength."

"Mercy killing" might well have been appropriate for "a demented animal". It did not even have to be considered for a "calm human being".

Much of what follows is based on an Address entitled "Moral problems facing the medical profession at the present time", written by the late Lord Bishop of Durham, Ian Ramsey, and read at the Annual Clinical Meeting of the British Medical Association in April 1972. Bishop Ramsey wrote:

"What has happened is that certain situations which are in outline what they have always been, have now changed radically in detail. For instance, medical treatment to save and prolong life; the need and the duty to ease pain; the conception and birth of a child; these are all situations which, overall and in outline, are the same as they have always been."

"Situations may be the same in outline—and therefore be supposed to yield broadly to traditional morality, and more particularly to the traditional code of professional behaviour. But their detail is infinitely more complicated, and this means that the old rules for dealing with these situations are far too large-scale to do justice to the new detail. It is as though we tried to catch sprats in the net of a trawler!"

The Bishop suggested that if we looked back at medical papers written in simpler times we might filter out such pre-suppositions, implicit as well as explicit, as those that follow: that life must be preserved; that patients have a right to control their own lives; that comparisons can be made between different people's lives in terms of quality; that medical research should proceed unhindered; that suffering must be avoided; that death is failure. In a series of logical (and acceptable) moves the Bishop, starting with that most commonly cited medical-moral principle "respect for life" enlarges this concept to "respect for human life in society at large". This is a fascinating and fundamental progress. The social dimension—family and society at large—is neglected at our peril. None of us is an island and we do not adequately respect a person's life unless we respect the lives of those other people who have constituted the community in which his life has been largely lived, and in which it has developed.

Having considered the principle of "respect for human life in society" Bishop Ramsey then points out that, closely connected with such problems as organ transplants, kidney machines or highly artificial means of keeping people alive, we are forced to see that what matters about life is not only or importantly its duration, but its value. So the original principle must be further expanded to read "respect for human life of a certain quality in society". Situations will and do arise when judgements will have to be made about the quality, and the potential quality, of one man's life against that of another. With one kidney machine available and needed, how should one, for example, judge between the value or the potential value, of a doctor and a Lord Justice? We know some people who are unquestionably dead; equally we know some people who are undoubtedly alive. But immediately one brings in a continuum, though it may be easy to see differences at the extremes, in the middle it is more difficult.

Case History

A woman with melanomatosis tried to commit suicide by throwing herself out of a window: she failed to kill herself. In the terminal stage of the disease she became our patient. She told us that after the suicide attempt one of her teenage children said, "You can't have loved us very much if you wanted so badly to leave us." Because she did live out her life to the full that family is now managing well.

One of the strongest arguments against euthanasia is the good use that patients and their families can make of the time after the pains have been controlled and before death finally occurs. To be denied such a time by an act of "mercy killing", instead of relying on good medical practice to alleviate the ills, would be to deprive the family, and society, of that unique value that is concentrated in any human life.

Is good medical practice in this field universally available? Unfortunately not. But that is not all the answer. Centres like St. Christopher's are being built, and prayed for (and fought for) all over this country, and indeed are spreading over the world. Variations on the theme of hospice care have been established and are working, not only as separate units or in the domiciliary field, but also within big hospitals, either as a special ward or as a team of specialists—doctors, nurses, social workers, chaplain—available for consultation whenever and wherever the pains of incurable disease call for the special skills that such a team possesses. A team of this kind began work at St. Thomas' Hospital, London, in January 1978.

Case History

At the 800-bedded St. Luke's Hospital, New York, they have set up what could be described as a symptom control team: two doctors, two nurses, a social worker and a chaplain, available for consultation throughout the hospital in any problem associated with terminal illness. Visiting there I was asked to see Robert. Arriving on the ward with the team we were greeted by the ward staff with, "We've certainly got problems with him." Robert had an osteogenic sarcoma with gross involvement of the left femur and hip. He was 23, black, an ex-Vietnam soldier, with a white girlfriend who was pregnant. His own parents would not visit him. He was on maximum doses of methadone (incorrectly administered), he was sweating with pain, unable to put a foot on the ground, and desperate. I doubt that a doctor had dared to touch him for several weeks. After shaking his hand and examining him I assured him that his pain could be controlled. The team (of which I was a temporary and honorary member) then went to consult with his doctors and the ward staff.

By rationalising his analgesics and adding phenylbutazone for the bony component of his pain and steroids for the inflammatory component, we enabled Robert to walk within 2 days. In a week he was able to walk out of the hospital to attend his father's funeral in North Carolina. He had to be readmitted within a month, and he died a few weeks later. Those who knew him well wrote: "Colour, education, class distinctions faded away in the face of courage and humility. There was acceptance at the end—a willingness to have it go either way. His concern was not for himself but for those who were closest to him."

I saw Robert for 20 minutes. I cannot recall ever seeing anyone for whom mercy killing would have seemed more appropriate. For Robert and those around him how good it was that he lived to the full the life that was left.

Conclusion

No new definition of "mercy killing" will get round the basic truth that *mercy is good but killing is bad*. What is needed is not more law, but codes of practice worked over by trans-disciplinary groups (not committees) functioning in the same sort of way that St. Christopher's are beating out a code of practice in the good use of narcotics for the relief of pain. Perhaps the Royal Colleges should be working on codes which involve not only the doctor and the nurse, but also the social worker and the chaplain, and which do not stop there: the most important yardstick for the success of such a venture is the involvement, trust and peace of mind of the patient and his family.

This, thank God, we repeatedly achieve and see achieved in ever-widening circles.

A new offence "mercy killing", would achieve nothing except to drive a further wedge of distrust between all parties involved. The ills for which "mercy killing" might be prescribed (that word is used advisedly—what starts off as a possibility will only too easily be turned into a duty) can almost always be alleviated by skill and compassion. The skills are available; therefore neither will the motives have to be judged nor the compassion be measured. Expertise does not have to give way to expediency.

10. DYING

Extract from On Dying Well, *Church of England Board for Social Responsibility**

I

No discussion of voluntary euthanasia would, or should, carry conviction, if it failed to take seriously the human realities of senility and death.

It is already being taught (*Amulree* 1969, *Fox* 1968, *Pilcher* 1967),[1] and frequently discussed in meetings of students and younger doctors (e.g. in such bodies as the London Medical Group and the society for the Study of Medical Ethics), that clinical judgement includes the responsibility of a doctor, in his pursuit of cure and of resuscitation, to decide at what stage it is in the real interests of a patient for him to step back and halt the process. His duty then is to relieve the pains of dying. It cannot be too strongly emphasized that this is a question of clinical duty, not one of law.

Moreover, just as the process of resuscitation is the work of a team, so too is the work of giving relief and peace to the mortally ill. In order to make these decisions and to give this relief, the doctor should consult with all who can provide relevant information concerning his patient. First among these are the family and nurses, who are the closest to the patient and who know him and the family, in most instances, far better than the doctor can. These consultations should include some attempt to discover the views of the patient himself. No statements made in the past by a patient can ever take the place of the patient's communication with his doctor. Good terminal care must include constant listening to the patient's own point of view, for a personal rapport is always of greater value than a piece of paper dating from an earlier time in the patient's life when he may well have had a different attitude.

What is appropriate treatment for one patient may well be inappropriate for another. No doctor claims that he will make infallible judgements, but that is no excuse for refusing to make decisions. "Curative" treatment is sometimes continued regardless of its relevance because no decision has been made. A family, who are pressing for "anything possible to be done", may not be told that the

*Reprinted by kind permission of the Central Board of Finance of the Church of England.

likely result of any further operation or treatment will merely prolong distress for the patient. The question is not "to treat or not to treat?" It is how to treat. To say that every active intervention possible must be pursued to the bitter end is as wrong and as heartless as to say, "There is nothing more to be done", and to abandon a patient. It is entirely misleading to call decisions to cease curative treatment "negative euthanasia"; they are a part of good medicine, and always have been.

Treating the Elderly

Much of the literature published about euthanasia concerns the elderly sick and expresses either fears that treatment will be pursued without regard for their wishes or the conviction that they are certain to end their days in long-stay geriatric units which may leave much to be desired. Further, on the one hand, complaints are heard about batteries of tests being inflicted on ill, elderly patients, and, on the other, there is often a negative or even nihilistic attitude to treating them at all. "But treatment, prognosis and planning for the patient's future is dependent on diagnostic accuracy." (*Agate*)[2] Requests to be allowed to die may be expressed in the course of an illness. However, modern geriatric methods, based on accurate diagnosis, frequently result in recovery, significant improvement, or the overcoming of major disabilities. When this happens it is the rule for patients to change their minds and no longer to express the wish to die. Many have acknowledged this change of heart and are grateful that their wish to die was not granted. The request to die should not be taken at its face value at the stage of an illness when morale is at its lowest and nursing and drug therapy have not had their chance. Consistent requests often stem from social conditions, and also from the feeling on the part of patients that they are now a burden upon those around them. The need for home support and the provision of help of all kinds (including financial assistance) for hard pressed families is often as great as that for medical treatment.

"There exists a very small minority of patients who have apparently decided for themselves that their time has come and that they now wish to depart. They seldom express it in words and they are not apparently confused, but their negative actions, refusal to eat or drink or to co-operate in any treatment, make their intention plain. It is usually pointless to try to prevent their behaving in this way and few geriatric physicians would seriously attempt to do so." (*Agate*, 1974).[3] These people, we note, do not say "Kill me"; their unexpressed wish is "Let me die". They can be, and commonly are, made comfortable if they become distressed or restless, and this leaves them free to change their minds at any time.

When potentially remediable illnesses occur in otherwise active old people, they should be treated actively. With diseases that have a poor prognosis it is questionable whether any except symptomatic treatment should be attempted. Once again accurate diagnosis is important in making this distinction. Elective operations of various kinds can be fully justified at almost any age for the relief of immobility, deformity, pain, discomfort or significant social disability. By contrast, the use of emergency resuscitation methods for cardiac arrest and other crises seldom seems justified in the elderly either on ethical grounds or on the results obtained. To discuss the question beforehand, with all who may be concerned, whether or not to resuscitate a given patient in the event of such a crisis, is preferable to setting a general age limit beyond which resuscitation should be withheld. All patients are different and these decisions must be individual and carefully arrived at. Most geriatric departments should be able to offer a high priority for admission to dying patients who need it. "There comes a time even in the most dramatic lethal illnesses when it is right finally to withdraw the life-support system, remove tubes, the infusion apparatus or oxygen mask and let the patient depart privately, peacefully and with dignity." (*Agate*, 1975).[4]

.Most people fear mental deterioration far more than they fear death. It is correct, although it may be small comfort, to inform those who fear greatly any loss of mental capacity that older people can and do adapt to changes in both mental and physical powers. Many disorientated and even demented people do not seem to be unhappy or distressed, and some are certainly quite the reverse. Insight into the change that is taking place is often lost at an early stage and, while this may seem to be a disaster in the eyes of the younger beholder, it is not so clear-cut a tragedy to the person concerned. Work with older patients reveals that, when prowess, activity and independence are diminished, life does not necessarily lose its meaning. A protected life, with sympathetic family or nurses (and there are more of both than some seem to think), may be a natural and acceptable sequel to life's activities. Even incontinence, the greatest dread of many, need be no more offensive nor humiliating at the end of life than it is at the beginning. It is certainly true that there are too many poorly housed and inadequately staffed long-stay units and too few good ones, but the answer to that is surely clear. It may also be emphasised that the more family and friends encourage independence and social importance, the less likely are mental powers to fail. "Senility" is sadly often a social disaster rather than an organic clinical condition and may be a retreat from isolation and unpleasant reality. To think merely in terms of easing such people out of life because of society's failure, would be to encourage still further the present tendency to seek easy and selfish ways out of all problems.

Anyone who has spent time with "senile" patients where they are lovingly cared for has seen how often they have much love both to give to, and evoke from, those who care for them. The happiness of such wards, not unlike that of some communities for the mentally handicapped, has an important perspective to offer to a society preoccupied with materialism and an over-intellectual approach to life.

Life Before Death

Life Before Death (*Cartwright et al.* 1973)[5] is a study which gives a picture of the way our society cared for a group of people, many of whom were sick for most of the year before their death, although it included a small number who had died suddenly without any previous illness.

It is based upon interviews with relatives and friends of 785 people, a random sample of adults who had died, and it was carried out in several selected areas in England. It is the fullest survey of this kind that has been carried out and tells us more of how people are in fact dying than anything that has been attempted before. It bears out what has been suggested in previous, smaller studies (*Aitken Swan* 1959, *Marie Curie Foundation* 1952, *Rees* 1972, *Wilkes* 1965).[6] Previous studies have concentrated upon cancer deaths; *Life Before Death*[7] has included all causes of death. In fact 20.6% died of cancer, 52.4% of various types of circulatory disease (including coronary artery occlusion and cerebral vascular accidents) and 14.8% of respiratory illness. Three-quarters of them needed some help during the last year of their lives, and most of their care devolved on relatives and friends.

This work revealed many gaps in the services and showed that there were insufficient beds in hospitals or appropriate homes, particularly for old people needing long term nursing care. The Community Services were often found to be deficient; for example, "nearly two-thirds of the district nurses felt that they would like to be able to give more time to those with terminal illness". The Home Help Service was not sufficiently staffed to give all the assistance that was needed, and housing for the elderly and sick at home was often unsatisfactory. Investment in these services by local government would mean death with decent dignity.

The study revealed loopholes and gaps in the co-ordination of the services, difficulties concerning admission to and discharge from hospital and failure of communication. Much may be hoped from the re-organization of services. A process which has been accelerated since the survey was finished. But we should all be deeply disturbed about the need which has been revealed in such careful detail.

One of the study's most disconcerting findings was the high

proportion of symptoms for which apparently no one had been consulted. Over half of those suffering from an offensive smell and of those with loss of bladder but not bowel control were said not to have sought help from any professional person even though the doctor was visiting. On the other hand, in spite of the heavy care often involved, it is heartening to read about the volume and intensity of care given by relatives and friends to many of those who had died. Much of the last year for most of the group was spent at home, and 40% died there. 59% of these people were aged 70 or over and there can be no doubt from these figures that families are still prepared to go to great lengths to care for those who are dying. Many still guard their independence and do not wish for outside help. This can never be forced on anyone, but, even so, continued independence with added community support should have been offered as an option. They should at least have been told what help was available.

Pain Control

Successful pain control is possible for many more patients than are yet receiving it. It could be widespread and it is already being taught extensively, but it has not yet reached far enough. 27% of spouses, where the patient had died at home, reported that the patient had severe pain which was given inadequate relief. A hospice is now operating a home-care programme in this district and is being called upon frequently for advice in pain control and for support for the family. Informal discussions and occasional conferences are also held with the local family doctors and district nurses. Similar programmes are developing in other districts, in most cases based on a hospice or similar home.

Thus the scene is gradually changing. More facts, such as those quoted above, are becoming available, more money has been allocated for the aged and chronically sick, and the reorganization of the community services is beginning to fill some of the gaps which have been revealed. It is to this process of fact-finding and consequent improvement of practical care and help that effort and attention should be directed if the large number of people known to suffer in their dying are to be reached and relieved.

Voluntary Euthanasia Irrelevant

At the same time, these studies suggest[8] that a law to legalise voluntary euthanasia would reach little of this distress. It would appear indeed that for most of the people concerned the effect would be adverse, directing attention away from their real needs and, more likely than not, making them feel a social pressure to think of themselves as unwanted citizens. It is not always recognized for how few people at present this question is of any relevance. Only a small proportion of the population plan ahead for their deaths to the extent of making a will. People are surely just as unlikely to set about signing forms of the kind that is suggested, unless some form of pressure were to be put upon them. The relatives questioned in the Parkes survey[9] were not asked their views on euthanasia, but in what were often long interviews they had ample opportunities to express any views they might have had. The interviewer who carried out the work reports that only one or two in the survey mentioned the matter at all. "It is fair to say that it did not appear to be a live issue for them."[10]

Medical provision is to a large extent a reflection of general social concern and it is important that the general public should be adequately informed and reminded of their responsibilities as members of a community which includes the weak and handicapped as well as the active and productive. Many of the families approached in the survey experienced little interest or help from anyone outside their immediate circle. Gorer has reported the isolation of the bereaved (*Gorer*, 1965).[11] Yet, in spite of general indifference, it is not difficult to arouse understanding and even action in an individual's particular situation. It is important that people should both be informed of need and be encouraged to respond to it.

Fears of Inevitable Pain should be Unjustified

It would seem just as important that they should know that proper care and support could achieve a gentle, dignified death for all, and that fears of inevitable pain should be unjustified. If every broadcast programme and every article in the press on the subject of death and dying could concentrate on the need for still more widespread provision of the kind of care that is increasingly available, rather than upon the call for voluntary euthanasia, it would do much to help the great majority. All of us are going to die. Confidence that such provision will be there when the time comes will be enough to reassure most people, who in any case prefer not to look towards their death and are unlikely to sign any forms concerning it.

If such care were always available, it is likely that some of those who do wish their deaths to be hastened would feel like the patient referred to in a letter recently received at a hospice: "X found real friends, real peace and real happiness during his last weeks, and his wife, while gratefully handing over the immediate responsibilities of his care and comfort, always felt fully involved and never isolated during his hospitalisation. I think you might be interested to hear that, as a friend and a member of the medical profession, I saw him become once more his old relaxed self with you and achieving your objective of alertness with minimal pain. During one of the many long talks we had peacefully in the ward he told me he had quite reversed his ideas on euthanasia—not because he was now near death and clinging to life from fear—but because he considered himself and his wife fortunate to bring life to a close in a dignified way and to be able to say those things that otherwise might have been left unsaid."

As another patient put it, "When I was in the teaching hospital I was acutely uncomfortable and could hardly bear myself at all, and I asked various friends of mine who were doctors if they would help me if I wanted to die and whether they would give me something, and a couple of them said Yes; but fortunately I never did ask for it. I think that fairly soon afterwards I heard that I was coming here, and it seemed to relieve the necessity. In a way I think I'm a very good argument against euthanasia. If I had accepted it I would have missed many weeks of really enjoyable life. I should hate to have done that."

II

Medical Education

In the book *Life Before Death*[11] a plea for changes in medical education and orientation is made. Only 2% of the sample surveyed in this study had died in teaching hospitals. "This suggests that not only are doctors rarely confronted with death during their training, but also that they do not see much of the illnesses which cause death . . . The skills inculcated and admired are diagnosis and specific therapy. Yet the common medical needs today are for the relief of chronic and common conditions."[12]

It is indeed no wonder that the doctor so often feels helpless and awkward in this situation and only stays briefly at the bedside of the dying patient, thinking that there is nothing he can do. And yet it can be shown daily in active geriatric units, in centres for terminal care and in homes visited by experienced family doctors, that it is possible to set out to diagnose and treat the causes of distress in incurable conditions and to apply specific therapy to relieve them.

A great deal of work has been carried out over recent years which has shown that distress can be relieved, both in hospital and in the patient's own home (*Hinton* 1967, *Lamerton* 1973, *Ross* 1970, *Saunders* 1963, 1964, in press).[13] Previously a neglected subject, the treatment of chronic and terminal pain is being considered, written of and taught (*Hart* 1974).[14] One hospice which has a teaching department, sends staff out to give nearly 200 lectures and talks in a year and welcomes some 2,000 visitors and nearly 100 residents, usually in multi-disciplinary groups. Another has had visits from 400 medical students in a year. Others have regular teaching sessions for the students in medical schools. Many post-graduate centres, local

77

medical societies and refresher courses in all disciplines concerned, all over the country, deal with this subject regularly. A section on "drugs for the dying" has for several years appeared in one of the textbooks of pharmacology (*Lawrence* 1966).[15] Terminal care is at last becoming part of a medical teaching and this subject recurs in many lectures and conferences organized by students themselves (see the programme of the London Medical Group).

Research is confirming that patients do not have to wait until their last hours for the relief of a dose of morphine, but that narcotic drugs can be used for months without detriment to the patient's personality or even activities (*Twycross* 1974).[16]

This is not "protracted euthanasia", or even a "living death", as it has been called, but a way of enabling someone to live actively up to the moment of his death. There are many other, less powerful drugs, and many ways of controlling pain, both for the patients with cancer (the disease most commonly mentioned in the euthanasia literature) and for those with other diseases which can also cause great and prolonged distress. There is also much knowledge concerning the control of other symptoms, including nausea, vomiting, breathlessness and depression. Technical resourcefulness can be combined with awareness of the individual patient's emotional and social needs and those of his family.

Misapprehensions

There are many misapprehensions concerning terminal pain and its relief. The general public fear that the pain in incurable illness, particularly cancer, is inevitable and cannot be relieved. Much has been made of this in the euthanasia literature. It is said that depressed consciousness must always accompany adequate relief and that strong analgesics (pain controlling drugs) have a decreasing effectiveness. The dangers of drug dependence (addiction) are feared by professional workers as well as by the public. Many appear to believe that a patient with terminal pain will need escalating doses of any drug used to relieve it and that this itself will eventually kill him. This has been described as "protracted euthanasia". It is implied that many doctors practise this already as their only alternative.

These fears must be allayed; for in fact the pain of terminal cancer can be fully relieved. In most cases effective drugs, available to any practitioner, can be given by mouth throughout a patient's illness. For a few patients drugs will have to be given by injection and usually these will be required for a short time only. All these drugs should be given regularly as routine medication and will prevent pain from occurring at all. This can be so for all but a very small number of cases. The patient will then not make his pain worse by his fear and tension and does not have to keep asking for relief. An ever-increasing number of drugs are also available to enhance the action of analgesics or, just as important, to treat other symptoms. They can be used in combination with analgesics. Records of large groups of patients treated at home as well as in hospital have shown that for the majority small doses of analgesics remain effective and that, where a large dose is required, it does not lose its effect nor does it necessarily depress consciousness. There is no "routine" dose. There is only the constantly reassessed dose for each individual patient who can in this way be given relief to the end of his life. Giving the right drugs correctly is not tantamount to killing a patient slowly. The relief of pain itself may well lengthen life: it will certainly enhance it.

Hospital Teams

It may be difficult, but it has been shown that it is not impossible, to do this in a general hospital ward; and a most welcome trend is the interchange and discussion which are being developed between teaching hospitals and hospices. Allied to this interest in several areas in the United Kingdom is the setting up of either a part of a hospital or of a team with a special interest and experience in such work. There is now no excuse for the unrelieved distress that is reported. Those who despair of giving relief and think that pain in inevitable should come and see what is being done.

A terminal illness can be transformed into a time for which everyone concerned is grateful. As the mother of a 21-year old put in a letter, "At one time during S.'s illness when he was desperately ill in hospital and in great agony, my only thought and prayer was that he should be spared further suffering; and I think I even actively wanted him to die, to be at peace, his agony was so terrible to see, and so little was done to relieve him. I know that, if anyone had told me then they could give him an injection which would end his pain, and also his life, I would have been tempted to say 'yes'. But I know we would have been wrong. It was soon after this that we came into contact with you and were able to fight with knowledge for what we knew was right for him. He did have pain again but not so terrible, and during those last four months he found a marvellous calm and acceptance, and the grace of God led him to a peaceful end which was an example to all who knew him. It has convinced me that it is never right to take a life—we do not know how God will work in what time is left."

If students are to learn something of the problem of illness in other than purely technical terms they need to be encouraged to work as members of interdisciplinary teams. The care for a dying person and his family must be a shared work and involves the nurses, the social workers and the chaplain; perhaps also the volunteer, the ward orderly and the receptionist. Any one of them may assume greater importance than the doctor for a particular family, for he is not automatically the leader of the team in every situation. Experience for students of various disciplines to work together during their training, and participation in formal and informal case discussions, important as they are in every branch of medical care, are essential in this field. Such a team will soon find that the family, the patient himself (and often other patients in the ward), and the workers of the relevant community services are also part of the group.

It has been noted that few families talk directly with dying patients about their illness. This may lead to much sorrow and bitterness after bereavement (*Parkes* 1970)[17] and it is important that the clinician should learn to listen to what the patient and his family are struggling, often incoherently, to tell him about their predicament. Much painful effort may be required in order to move from an entrenched position of denial to one where the fatal illness can be directly faced. As it is, people are left alone with the very truth from which everyone around them is persuading himself they are being protected, and even the family doctor does not find it easy to reach a position of mutual frankness with a patient or his family. Here again the team is important. Both family and patient are likely to speak of their anxieties with the nurses, the students, the junior doctors, in fact everyone before they are able (if they ever are) to speak to the consultant who never appears without his entourage. Progress in real meeting may be made if the other members of the team can be encouraged to share information with the doctor who has the final responsibility for giving it to the patient.

Patients do not criticize doctors who try to open up communication on the subject of mortal illness (*Hinton* 1974),[18] and much mental pain is eased when doctors learn how to listen.

We do not know where the consequences of legislation permitting voluntary euthanasia would end; we do know that possibilities of relief already exist. Research and planning in this whole field and, above all, teaching for all the professions involved are called for if people are to die more easily and with greater dignity.

Relief Available to All

The positive medical approach is to work for this and at the same time see that everything possible is done to ease the passage of the "hard cases" now and in the future (when there should be many fewer of them). Those who believe that any legislation in this area would lead to an unpredictable amount of suffering, and almost certainly much abuse, have a responsibility to work towards a situation in which no one should ever have to ask for release because of unrelieved distress. It has been shown that this is possible; the thrust is now to make relief available to all.

Notes

1. S. Amulree, "James Mackenzie and the future of Medicine", *Journal of the Royal College of General Practitioners*, Vol. 17, p. 3, 1969.
   T. R. Fox, "Purpose of Medicine", *Lancet*, Vol. 2, 1965, p. 801.
   R. S. Pilcher, *Valedictory Address on his retirement from the Professorship of Surgery at University Hospital Medical School*, 1967.
2. J. Agate, "Ethical Considerations: How far Does One Go?" from *Modern Medical Treatment*, ed. H. Miller and R. Hall, 1975.
3. J. Agate, *Personal Communication*, 1974.
4. J. Agate, *Op. Cit.* 2. above.
5. A. Cartwright, L. Hockey, J. L. Anderson, *Life Before Death*, Routledge & Kegan Paul, 1973, London and Boston.
6. J. Aitken-Swan, "Nursing the late cancer patient at home", *Practitioner*, Vol. 183, p. 64, 1959; Marie Curie Memorial Foundation, *Report on a National Survey Concerning Patients with Cancer Nursed at Home*, 1952; W. D. Rees, "The Distress of Dying", *British Medical Journal*, Vol. 2, p. 105, 1972; E. Wilkes, "Terminal Cancer at Home", *Lancet*, Vol. 1, 1965, p. 799.
7. *Op. Cit.*, 5. above.
8. See also the paper by Dr. T. West *P.*
9. C. M. Parkes, *Personal Communication*, 1974.
10. *Ibid.*
11. *Op. Cit.* 5. above.
12. *Ibid.*
13. J. Hinton, *Dying*, Penguin Books Ltd, 1957; R. Lamerton, *Care of the Dying*, Priory Press, 1979; E. Kubler-Ross, *On Death and Dying*, Tavistock Publications, 1970; C. M. Saunders, "Treatment of intractable pain and terminal cancer", *Proceedings of the Royal Society of Medicine*, Vol. 55, p. 191, 1963; C. M. Saunders, "The Symptomatic treatment of incurable malignant disease", *Prescribers Journal*, Vol. 4, p. 68, 1964; C. M. Saunders, "Terminal Care", *Medical Oncology*, Ed. K. D. Bagshawe, Blackwell, 1975.
14. F. D. Hart, *The Treatment of Chronic Pain*, Medical & Technical Publishing Co., 1974.
15. D. R. Lawrence, *Clinical Pharmacology*, 3rd Edition, J. & A. Churchill, 1966.
16. R. G. Twycross, "Clinical experience with diamorphine in advanced malignant disease", *International Journal of Clinical Pharmacology, Therapy and Toxicology*, Vol. 9, p. 184, 1974.
17. C. M. Parkes, "The first year of bereavement", *Psychiatry*, Vol. 33, p. 444, 1970.
18. T. Hinton, "Talking with people about to die", *British Medical Journal*, Vol. 2, p. 25, 1974.

11. DISCIPLINE OF THE CROSS

Group Captain Leonard Cheshire V.C. D.S.O. D.F.C.

I find the title "Discipline of the Cross" is very meaningful and a very thought provoking one, in fact I think it's the first time that I have seen those two words put together—the Discipline of the Cross. And I have to admit that it has caused me to sit and think about the particular relevance of their juxtaposition. And as I think, it's better that anything I say, comes out of my own experience, rather than an attempt to be speculative, I would like to confine myself mainly to disabled people; in other words the problems of disability, and perhaps also the dying—to the meaning of death.

Masterpieces Fashioned by God

In order to say anything about the Cross, and to give it any meaning at all, we need to consider what is our purpose in life? Where is it we are aiming to go? If we are not clear about that, it's difficult to see how we can put any major element of our life, or our journey through this world, into perspective. Obviously there are many ways, and from different points of view, one could attempt to define man's purpose and destiny on earth. The way I would like to put it, is this; that our purpose as individuals, you and me, and everybody else, members of the one human family, is to build ourselves into the unique masterpiece that God intends for each one of us. Each of us unique and each of us to be a masterpiece. That is what God wants of us.

I think the simile of the potter from Jeremiah (8:1–10) is a very good simile for our purposes. What distinguishes Man from every other living being in creation is that Man is both nature—and person. Our nature in which we all share (I suppose some more fortunately than others) might be compared to the clay that the potter uses, and our person to the potter. Each of us in life has to work on that little bit of human nature which is ours, which is mine, with its defects and its grandeur and mould it into a masterpeice. But that's not all. Because we don't stand just as individuals, we stand as members of the one human family, and what God intends for each of us, He also intends, in a different order, for the entire human family. He intends, as we all believe as Christians, that the human family will itself ultimately become a perfect and unique masterpiece in its own right, an integrated being with Christ Our Lord the Head and we His members. So that we are here on earth not just to perfect ourselves, which of course we can only do if God is allowed to lead us, but to play our part in bringing the entire human family to ultimate perfection.

I would go so far as to say that even that isn't all, that God's plan, so movingly described in St Paul's letter to the Ephesians, God's plan for the fullness of time is to unite all things in Christ, things on earth with things in heaven. The Church tells us in the Liturgy that it's the whole of creation that is to be brought into a unity, and that everything that we do on earth, provided it's good and morally upright, is in fact building eternity. Our human relationships, our work, everything that we do has a good and right purpose, is in fact, constructing eternity. Ultimately, I believe we will carry through with us into our eternal home, the works of our hands, the works of our daily lives, to be eternalised, divinized by the power of God's Holy Spirit. So in that context where do we see the place of the cross?

If we look first at those who are disabled and ask ourselves, if we can, what is the meaning of disability?[1] What role has disability to play, not only in the lives of those whom it has struck, but the rest of us who are able-bodied, who have not been through that experience.

I think I need to start by making just two statements about disability so that we know what we are talking about. There is a tendency in life I find, for all of us to put labels round people's necks. We label people into groups and then we think we know who they are. For instance, we have a tendency to talk about "the disabled" as if they formed a separate group different from the rest of us, and of course that is wrong. A disabled person is first and foremost and fundamentally a person, and only incidentally someone who has a disability. And the term disability itself; what does it mean? Usually I know we use it to indicate somebody who is physically handicapped but its real meaning is an impairment of any one of our faculties, whether physical, mental or emotional. So that means that if I for instance, have a personality defect—which means that I can't cope with a normal social situation that other people can cope with—I have a disability. If for instance, once launched upon a talk or a lecture, I am completely unable to bring it to an end, you'd probably say (I don't know how politely) "that man isn't quite normal!" Now I know we can't push this point too far, but I make it in order to establish a basic truth that the borderline between disability and non-disability, or whatever the term is, is a very fine one. All of us have our many shortcomings and we should be very careful before we put the disabled person in a different category of his own, unless of course we are doing it for a medical or other professional purpose, that is different.

Now I'd like to look also at the personal side of disability. What does it mean to the human being to be struck by disability, to become either suddenly or gradually severely disabled? And also, what is it that the disabled person wants? What is his basic role in life and how can we help him towards it? Usually the goal of the disabled person, the goal which we should be aiming at, when we set out to help disabled people, or rather share their struggle is to find independence, and it's said that the greater independence you can give the disabled person the nearer you approach the goal.

I used to think that too, and I used that in talks I gave. More latterly on reflecting on it, I've begun to think that isn't correctly expressed, it's not correctly defined. Because, after all, there is not a single one of us who is really independent—we are all interdependent. The very fact that we are common members of the one human family means that we are social beings. We are not created to live on our own and every single day each of us is dependent upon all kinds of help and services from other people. To push independence too far would risk becoming arrogant. So although helping somebody to greater independence is clearly essential, I don't believe that is a correct definition of our goal.

I think a better definition is freedom. Freedom to choose the kind of life that he or she wants. That seems to me to lie at the heart of the whole Christian view of life; the whole history of salvation—that we are free beings, and because free, responsible. And so what society should provide, or aim to provide for disabled people, is a whole range of different living facilities and different forms for help in the way of aids and gadgets so that each person can decide what he wants. I know some people who get quite dogmatic on the subject. They say that every disabled person should have this and not have that and so on, but I find that every disabled person is different, quite different from the next. And there is not such a thing as an ideal solution. Some people say you should have residential homes, that is putting disabled people separate from the community. I know many disabled people who actually want the community life. I know many able-bodied people who choose community life because they find that it gives them something that living on their own does not. So I think we should be very careful before we over-generalise about the needs of the disabled person.

What is it that the disability means to him, in his heart? That is what I'd like to try and look at. I'd like to try if I can, though I hope it's not presumptuous to look inside the heart of somebody, particularly somebody young who has become suddenly severely disabled (because then it's the hardest to accept). Perhaps on an afternoon swim, diving into water that's too shallow and breaking their neck. That person becomes severely handicapped—a tetraplegic. To begin with he probably goes to an intensive care unit and there there is an atmosphere of efficiency, there are doctors, there are specialists, there are machines. Everything is so purposeful and you feel that despite what it looks like, it's not going to be quite so bad as it appears. There is hope. But then—the moment will come when you are perhaps moved to a general ward or back home, or to some other form of institution, and there in some way or another, somebody will say to you that you are never going to get any better. He may say it very gently. It may take him nearly a week to say it—but that is what he is telling you—you will never get any better.

Now what happens inside the heart of somebody—perhaps a 19 year old—ready to launch out into life, suddenly finding that nothing she ever wanted to do is going to be possible. I think first there is a sense of grief, of mourning. You mourn for what you have lost in the same way that we mourn the loss of somebody very close to us. I think that the sense of mourning may last a person's entire life even if it's just deep down inside their being. But it is soon followed by something quite different, something that I can only call a revolt. You actually rebel; you say to yourself, "Why?—Why has this got to happen to me, why now, just at this moment when everything was opening up for me?" You even find people who blaspheme, they throw away their faith, they may say all kinds of things. Now what should be our reaction? What should we do to help that person, assuming that we are close to them? The worst thing we can do is to ignore it, to pretend it isn't there. What we have to do is to grasp it, we somehow have to help that person work it out of their system. I think the only way we can do that is by giving them time. We have to give time, to be with them and build up a relationship in which they feel secure. That is to say, they feel they can say anything they like, however dreadful it may sound, knowing that they won't be judged. If they think they are going to be judged they'll never say it, but if they can once say it, then gradually it will work out of themselves and then they can begin to build a whole new life.

I am sure you will know in your contacts with disabled people that the hall-mark of those who are disabled is cheerfulness, purposefulness, normality. You see them looking so cheerful, so concentrating on what they can give tomorrow, that perhaps we overlook that deep inner struggle that they have had to go through. Of course that struggle has given them a character and a strength that perhaps we who may not have been through a struggle don't have. I don't believe it is possible to achieve depth and strength of character and real compassion for other people without going through some measure of struggle or difficulty of one kind or another.

The other problem that the disabled person faces, (I think we will all agree, that it is one of our basic needs as a human being) is to feel valued. We want to feel that other people value us for something we have actually done. Perhaps it may just be having been a very good mother of a family, having had a very good relationship with one's family, or it may be an achievement in some area of work. We also have a need at a much deeper level of our being, to be valued for the person we are, not valued for the person we ought to be. If we find that we are accepted by other people for what they like in us, we aren't really secure. I want to feel that people will accept me for what I am and this is the way that God deals with us. God loves us not for anything good that we have done, but because He loves us, and the patience which He shows with our shortcomings, with our broken resolutions, is to me almost incomprehensible, but it makes us feel secure, it makes us feel that we are wanted, and on our side we know how difficult it is to accept others for the person they actually are. We are always wanting them to become the person we think they should be, and with the disabled person who now suddenly feels that he will never achieve anything for which he will be admired, this is a very great problem.

Today with the advance of technology I think you can say that nobody, however disabled, is not able to lead a purposeful and constructive life given the right environment and given the right aids. You only have to look at the life of a girl—Hilary Pole—you may have read or know of her. A young girl who became completely paralysed to a point where she couldn't breathe, she couldn't see, she couldn't talk and she could move no part of her body except one big toe on her right foot. She was given a breathing machine, she was artificially fed and then somebody designed an electronic box which was operated by a little microswitch on a board that was fitted to her right foot. Through this, apart from being able to put on her hi-fi, for she was very musical, she could type, and you would go to Hilary, talk to her, for she could hear although she couldn't see you, and she'd answer back on her typewriter; a kind of little shorthand typing that she did. Apart from that she spent her time organising appeals to raise money for other disabled people to have equipment they hadn't got, writing poetry and also counselling other disabled people if they felt they didn't know how to cope. They'd write to her or go and see her and she would counsel them—she'd help them overcome their problems. Now that was Hilary's life up to her death about 4 years ago. In all truthfulness, a beautiful life, a life of such purpose and determination. I know there are some people who would say, and one has to respect their sincerity, well if that's her condition, wouldn't it have been better just to let her slip away. But Hilary was determined to live and to make something out of her life and that is how she did it. And I think that the example she and practically all other disabled people, amongst whom I would include the very poor of the world, the lonely, and all others who are under-privileged in one way or another, poses the question for us: what is the true criterion of human achievement? Is it the achievement itself or is it what we have put into it?

And you remember the moment when Our Lord was sitting in the temple and people were putting their money in the collection box and He looked at an old lady and said, "That widow with her farthing", whatever it was worth, "has given more than the wealthy with their big gifts, because they have given out of their wealth and she has given everything that she had."[2] The way He said that, is clearly not a parable. He was telling us we have to believe the truth, that her gift was bigger than theirs. I know that's very difficult to believe but I think that it shows us that the only way you can really measure the true value of any contribution, is in relation to the person's opportunities and resources. That seems to be the way God assesses achievement, and that means there is nothing in life that is not something that can be put to value, to good use. It means that there is nobody, however poor, however helpless, who in fact is not able to contribute to our divinely given destiny of building up to the full stature of perfection. Building up to that unique masterpiece that God wants each of us to be and building the entire human family. And somehow to me that alters everything, because it's so easy to feel that everything is pointless, we feel we have achieved nothing, we long to be in a situation where we can get results, and if we can only hold on to the conviction, the faith that so long as we play our part God will give a meaning and a purpose to everything. In fact to me, the most important thing in life, humanly speaking, is that we should always be in that place where God wants us, and then do our best according to the circumstances of the moment.

The discipline of the Cross as I see it, really means the obedience of the Cross. If we look at Our Lord and look at His life, not only do we constantly hear Him say I've come not to do My will, but the will of Him who sent Me. He also put it differently: He said, "The words I speak are not My words they are my Father's words,"[3] and it is that which enabled Him to fulfil His life's mission. I think it's easy for us Christians to concentrate so much on the fact that Our Lord is the Son of God and divine, as to forget that He is also truly Man and that He had to go through everything in the same way that we have to go through it, and that must include discovering what His life's mission was and how He was to achieve it.

Lent commemorates the day when Jesus after His baptism was sent out by the Holy Spirit. The word I think really means in the Hebrew, pushed out into the desert for 40 days where He was tempted. Now I know of course, that those 40 days have immense significance and can be interpreted in many different ways, all of them correctly. But to me they have a special message. I think that the reason He had to spend those 40 days there was to learn from His Father how He was to carry out His life's mission. Because the way He did it in the end was contrary to all our human ways of reckoning. None of us would ever have imagined that the salvation of the world could have been brought about in the way that Jesus set about it. And I think, that during those 40 days, the essential struggle He was having to undergo and win, was accepting His Father's will as to how He was to achieve His mission.

All of us have to do that in our lives and I think we all discover during the course of our lives that suffering the Cross, in whatever form it comes, is a way of discipline, it's a way of compelling us to listen. Obedience, I think I'm right in saying, basically comes from listening—auscultare—listen. To listen and to hear God's will for us. In addition it was through the Cross and suffering that the Son of God chose to redeem the world and therefore whatever part we may share in suffering or in associating ourselves with somebody else's suffering, is a participation in the redemptive work of Christ, and I think to bring that theme to an end we must remember that death is an integral part of this lifelong process of lifting ourselves up towards perfection, towards the full stature of perfection that God intends for us. Death is not just a sudden ending of our life, it is not just a separation of soul and body, though that it is. In death, in its inner content, there is I am convinced, a struggle that deep down in the person, unseen by anybody else, known only to the person himself and God, is a struggle without which we can never achieve perfection. I believe that struggle to be essentially one of faith. We are called to be men of faith and of course in our lives we don't live up to that. But there still remains our dying, and I believe personally, that in our dying, we are going to be called to make the supreme act of faith in our lives, of our whole lives.

It is easy to think that if we have done our best to live a Christian life, then death is merely the gateway into our eternal home. Perhaps it is, but somehow it doesn't seem to measure up to what we see in the life and the dying of Our Lord. His dying was not only immensely painful, in His dying he felt a complete rejection. He cried out, "My God, My God, why has Thou forsaken Me?"[4] I do not believe that those words can be explained away as merely something for our benefit. If, as we know He did, He became sin for us, took upon Himself responsibility for all our faults, then He had to be at that moment (although it is difficult to even say) repugnant to His Father. His Father, if He really had become sin, would reject Him. And I think that it may be in our dying, at some moment in our dying, we also may feel abandoned. We may not be able to see God as a God of love, except by faith. We may be called to step out into the unknown, not knowing what is going to be the outcome, and I personally think that all of us should pray for that moment of death so that we won't fail, so that we will step out into the unknown in our final act of faith that will bring us, and in bringing us, will help carry over others to our eternal home. We've each come to live a particular life and to die a particular death, and in that living and in that dying, it is our task, to the best of our ability, to bring ourselves to perfection. If it seems difficult we can remember and hold on to the knowledge that we may sow the seed, and we may water, and we may weed and dig round, but it's God who gives the increase.[5]

That to me is the lesson of the Cross. That we hold on no matter what happens to us in our living and in our dying, to the knowledge that God will lift us up to be that final and unique masterpiece that He means for each of us.

Notes

1. See also John Steensma's paper p.39 and Dr. Koop's p.27.
2. Luke 21:1–4.
3. John 14:10.
4. Matt. 22:47.
5. Mark 4:26–9.

12. CONTINUING PROBLEMS ARISING FROM THE MONGOL BABY CASE, 7th OF AUGUST, 1981 (COURT OF APPEAL, LONDON)

V. E. Hartley Booth, LL.B.

A twelve-day old child, Alexandra, suffering from mongolism and an intestinal blockage, has created legal history. Whether she should receive an operation that might save her life was disputed. The parents argued it was kindest and best for the child to be allowed to die. The Local Authority and The Official Solicitor for the child, argued against it. It was mentioned in Court that adoptive parents were forthcoming. The result, the ordering of the operation is well known. This case has highlighted a number of medico and medico-legal, as well as Christian, points. Many have already been raised in this book.

As a lawyer, who this year is Chairman of a group of professional people including many of whom are doctors and lawyers and all Christian, I have been very much involved in the discussions. I attempt here to summarise various points in this debate, emphasising a few that have been buried, or forgotten. The points covered here include: the doctor's discretion, the role of the Court, whether nature should be allowed to take its course, the place of adoption and fostering, some further developments on this subject and the law and sanctity of life. Throughout this paper, it is an underlying theme that the distressed parents and the particular child deserve our greatest sympathy. I have tried to move away from referring to the particular case wherever possible.

Should the doctor's discretion be subject to the Court? Or is the court's role better seen as a useful arbitrator when exercise of discretion is difficult?

Doctors were quick to condemn the court as interfering in what they saw as parental and medical discretion alone. Jeremy Lawson (*Pulse*, Vol. 41. No. 33. August 13th 1981), Paediatric Surgeon, Westminster Children's Hospital, was reported to say, "I would not go ahead (to perform the operation) without the parents' consent. The decision of the Court of Appeal is going to make more difficult what we feel is the right decision." Professor John Lorber head of the department of paediatrics at the Children's Hospital, Sheffield said (*The Times* 13th

August) "The decision of the Court of Appeal was very, very wrong. It was against the interests of the parents, the child and society." But the medical profession was divided. The day before, on the 12th August, Professor R. B. Zachary also of the University of Sheffield summed up a widely felt view in writing in his letter to the *Daily Telegraph*, "In this year of the handicapped person let us not say, 'Abandon hope all you who are born mentally retarded.'" A G.P., Dr. Margaret White, said on the same day in *The Times*, "As the cousin of a mongol I was sad to see that though the Court of Appeal made the right decision in authorising life-saving surgery for a baby girl with Down's Syndrome, they did it for the wrong reason." The British Medical Association weighed in during the week after the decision saying through a spokesman, "A newborn baby has rights in the same way as any other patient. Normally the parent makes decisions on the child's behalf but in very rare circumstances the doctor may believe the decision should be taken out of the parent's hands."

The division of medical opinion was not only evident among the doctors who professionally considered Alexandra's case but the uncertainty led to the Court case. The Consultant Paediatrician at Queen Charlotte's Hospital for Women was of the view that, while sympathising with the feelings of the other doctors who had been consulted, the alternative course involved starving the child and possible sedation until death and was one he was not personally prepared to undertake. The doctors who were consulted in the Hospital for Sick Children, Great Ormond Street, took the view already expressed that the parents' attitude was more decisive.

All this confusion precisely illustrates the importance and the role of the Court. The law acted as the arbitrator. Far from the Court and local authority interfering both were called in to help. Both had no choice but a legal duty to act. It was the Queen Charlotte's doctors who approached the social workers to intervene and have a chat with the parents initially. The local authority made the child a ward of court. It was the Court that took the responsibility when medical discretion was uncertain and divided.

Whereas the doctors seeing distressed, articulate parents are bound to be mindful of the anguish an unfortunate couple is suffering they are also, as in this case, in the position of being the doctor in charge of an inarticulate patient a few days old.

By contrast the Court were able to hear separate representation for the child, through counsel instructed by The Official Solicitor, the parents and the potential foster parents or adoptive parents through the local authority solicitor respectively. The Court was in a position to be more objective. Society places huge burdens on the medical profession. It is unfair perhaps that so much should fall upon them unmitigated. It is also perhaps blinkered of some to view the help of the courts as interference.

A more fundamental question was asked by many. Is it wrong to interfere with natural events at all?

As asked, this question broadens the last point considerably. The scope of this question even queries the doctor's right to save a life which would otherwise extinguish itself by natural process. The consultant paediatrician at High Wycombe and Amersham Hospitals in Buckinghamshire, Dr. Donald Garrow, was reported in the *Daily Mail* (10th August) to say, "I think it is wrong and bad to interfere with natural events. Nature made one mistake and then it made another. The two mistakes together cancelled each other out and this child should have been allowed to die." He continued, "If you have a reasonable expectancy of a normal life, then most people must believe it is right to operate to save that life. If on the other hand there is no expectancy of a normal life then most people would believe that anything which ends that life is a merciful deliverance." *The Daily Telegraph* (8th August) reported that this argument was canvassed in Court. This newspaper recorded Roger Gray, Q.C., counsel for the parents, as stating, "God or Nature has given the child a way out and so the parents' wishes should be respected."

Ironically the weakness in this whole argument was exposed by Roger Gray himself. He was reported by the same source to say, "There is no evidence whether the child would be happier alive or dead. Nobody can tell what the sufferings of this little child will be if she is allowed to live." Nor, we are entitled to add, what happiness.

Of course the child, Alexandra, in this case was not able to give her views but Francis A. Schaeffer in Chapter II of *Whatever Happened to the Human Race* asked a number of severely handicapped people would they prefer to have died at birth. All preferred to live. Mary Moloney a 16 year old child with Down's Syndrome (*Daily Mail*, 10th August) beat her mother at tennis and her mother, Pauline, said, "She has certainly enriched our lives. She's absolutely marvellous and I think so every time I look at her." The cousin of Dr. White (*The Times*, 12th August) was a mongol who wrote an illuminating book entitled *The world of Nigel Hunt*. His principle point was the happiness that life meant to him.

Hugh Jolly, Physician in charge of the Paediatric Department, Charing Cross Hospital, London, in the third edition of his book, *Diseases of Children*, page 219 while accepting that "all mongols are mentally handicapped, the I.Q. usually lying between 35 and 55, very rarely the I.Q. may be as high as 70", stated that "most mongols are friendly and they often show an unusual enjoyment of music".

What are the parents' rights to allow or refuse an operation that might save a child's life?

The parent as the guardian at law of the child has power to act for the child's good and for its protection. The power includes some discretion but not as much discretion as an adult has over his or her own life. Thus for example although an adult may legally commit suicide (Suicide Act 1961) a parent may not kill a child in its care.

An operation may normally only be performed with the permission of the parents. The basis of this is that surgery may involve what might otherwise be an assault on the child. The Chancery Division of the English High Court has an ancient prerogative right of the Crown. The term used is parens patriae. The Court may agree to accept guardianship of an infant who is made a Ward of Court. Until the jurisdiction of the Court is invoked either under this prerogative or under Statute of which there are now several (see first, The Guardianship of Infants Act 1925 s.4) all parental rights and powers are vested in the father of a legitimate child under common law. When however a child has been made a Ward of Court, the Court assumes the powers of the parents. At that moment the parents lose these rights and in that sense are strangers to the child. They however may be represented personally in court by advocates. Technically they "intervene" in the wardship proceedings, this does not oust the powers of the Court but they can argue for the Court to exercise their powers in the way they want or they can argue for the wardship to be discharged. The Court has a duty to listen to these arguments.

The common law gave rights and the Court of Chancery declared duties. The Tenures Abolition Act 1660 summarised the common law rights of parents and guardians as the right to custody, tuition and management of the infant (including the right to determine his religious upbringing) and the right to manage his property. The Court declared that the father was bound to maintain his children (Fawkner v. Watts (1741) 1 Atk.408). Most lawyers would agree with the assertion in the letter of the Lawyers for the Defence of the Unborn (*Times* 17th August 1981) that a general principle exists that "parents are responsible for the wellbeing of their children and have a duty to consent to medical treatment which is likely to improve the child's health and life expectation." Nothing in the law specifically helps as to whether the quality of life is either relevant or predictable.

What regard can we or should we have to the future quality of life of a sick child?

The judges try to do their best. The Court of Appeal in the Mongol Baby case inferred that the quality of life was relevant. The judges agreed that there was no evidence that the little girl's life was likely to be an intolerable one. This was criticised by Dr. White (*The Times* 12th August) in a point taken by the Magazine *Doctor*, August 20th 1981. "Whether a baby can look forward to a good quality of life is something no one can predict." She wrote: "Most people would accept that the deaf and blind Helen Keller had a better quality of life than the rich and beautifully tragic Marilyn Monroe. The right of a baby girl to a life saving operation should not depend on her future intelligence quotient or facial appearance any more than it should on her race or sex."

On the other hand there is the much quoted maxim "Thou shalt not kill but needst not strive officiously to keep alive" (Arthur Hugh Clough: *The Latest Decalogue*). Most agree with this, including the *Guardian* 10th August and Ann Kent in *Pulse* August 22nd. There is however all the difference in the world between the way in which medicine was used to maintain the body of General Franco in weeks of limbo and doing a simple life saving operation to remove an intestinal blockage caused by duodenal atresia, analogous in complexity to an appendectomy, on a young mongol.

Professor Zachary writing in the *Telegraph*, 12th August 1981 put the logical side of the point most graphically, "Suppose that this child were now two or three years old and was with her parents in the park by the side of the paddling pool when she rolled or crawled and fell into the pool. Would it be right for the parents to stand idly by and watch the struggles of the child for two or three minutes? And if a passerby jumped into the pool and was about to lift out the child would the parents have the right to stop him saying: 'No she is a mongol, we are the parents and we do not give our consent'?"

What of the other side of the coin? It is often said the parents must look after the child. The years of difficulty they must experience must be allowed to weigh. Why should the parents be forced to look after a child in that state of health?

Every sympathy must go to the parents. The *Guardian* (10th August) put it sensitively. The agony of the parents must not be underestimated: "No-one should preach at the parents of a handicapped child: no-one should mistake their deep distress especially after the birth." But, as the *Guardian* continued, emotions must not override logic.

What is not mentioned except in passing in the press, though a reference was made to it in the Courts' judgement, was that "the local authority was confident that good adoption arrangements could be made to provide the child with a happy life". (*Times*, "Law Report" August 8th 1981).

The law provides for distressed parents who cannot cope with the situation that confronts them. The provision made is the process known as adoption. This does not cover the parents who suggest that the child is better dead but the facts about adoption should perhaps be better known.

Adoption has been part of English law since 1926. The Tomlin Committee described it as "a legal method of creating between a child and one who is not the natural parent of the child an artificial family relationship analagous to that of parent and child" (1925 Cmnd 2401). Hammersmith and many other local authorities have no difficulty placing children of any age and state of health with excellent parents. One small national adoption society has about twenty babies a year to place with parents. A thousand couples come forward. 980 couples are disappointed. Thanks to new methods of publicising the existence of Down's Syndrome and other children in need of adoption, they stand a better chance than ever before of being adopted (*Doctor*, August 20th 1981).

The underlying absurdity of this clamour was pointed out by Dr. Alan Shrank (*Times* 18th August 1981) that while "One in seven healthy foetuses are legally and unnaturally aborted mostly on social grounds, childless couples compete to adopt the handicapped".

The only child one well known local authority has ever had difficulty in placing for adoption was blind and deaf, coloured, crippled and aged 13. But a loving couple were found to care for him.

The alternative of foster parents is also often ignored. One radio programme included a remark, "How can the court and officials love a child better than the child's natural parents?" The question forgets that it is adoptive or foster parents that will be loving the child in nearly all cases wonderfully well.

It is hoped that the misconception held by many including a writer to the *Times* (14th August 1981), that a severely handicapped child rejected by his parents has no chance of adoption, can be corrected. One society has even gone into print to say so. "Parents for Children" wrote in the *Times* (25th August 1981), "In the last five years this agency alone has placed 22 mentally handicapped and 12 physically handicapped children for adoption."

The Future: What evidence?
The case of Alexandra was clear about one thing: if there had been

no operation, death would have resulted from starvation and that often such children are sedated to the point of death. The alternative was a straightforward operation with uncertain clinical prognosis.

It has also been asserted that because the cause lies in so fundamental a body structure as a chromosome, no cure or fundamental alleviation will be found. We all enjoy the benefit of a grandstand view of history, and have seen how cells, atoms, bacteria and viruses have fallen under the manipulation of scientists.

The only allusion in the Press to the medical advance in the treatment of Down's children was made by the Down's Society. It said (24th August 1981 *Times*) that changes in treatment of these children in recent years both in Europe and the United States have significantly improved their performance. Dr. Ruth H. Harrell in the *Proceedings of the National Academy of Sciences USA*, Vol 78, January 1981, reported work with Down's Syndrome children. The administration of large doses of vitamins at certain stages in their childhood resulted in marked improvements in appearance and intelligence. Already information sheets on the use of vitamins are being used by medical practitioners in the United Kingdom. Educational improvements and changes in attitude have similarly begun to significantly improve the Down's child's chances.

The advances in knowledge have come too late to help these mongol children, who have died in the mistaken belief that nothing could be done to improve their prognosis. They emphasise the fact that hope always exists for medical and social improvement. It is hoped that future mongol children will not suffer from this ignorance, but will be given the best possible chances to reach their potential, which is constantly increasing.

A fact also forgotten by certain doctors, who genuinely respect the parents' decision made at the hospital, was spoken about by the director of Hammersmith Social Services. He said (*Daily Telegraph* 11th August), "The birth of a handicapped child often throws parents into a trauma and they could make decisions they might regret later."

It was rightly stated in the case of Alexandra that a mongol child with an added handicap should be put in a position of any other mongol child, so far as possible.

The Law: The Sanctity of life and Right to live?
"You either believe life is sacred or you don't. Once you have decided, that is it. There is no argument on this matter. It is a matter of belief." So goes the argument. It is an emotive phrase to some, but has the advantage of explaining its own basis. It is implicit in the word "sacred" that God is involved. At once the origin of the belief is

understood even if not accepted. By contrast the phrase "right to live" used by many is a term which is confusing in a country where there is no written constitution granting such a right, no body of law explaining such a right nor legal method of enforcing the provision of life, especially if one takes the provider of life to be God. And the compromise used by many is the phrase "respect for life". This last however is equally confusing. "Respect" implies the notion of the "doffed cap" and the changing pattern of what is polite and what deserves respect. Sanctity has the advantage of being eternal and if we don't wear black top hats at funerals so often nevertheless life continues to be sacred!

Few lawyers have done more to de-sanctify this term than Professor Glanville Williams who wrote *The Sanctity of Life and the Criminal Law* in 1956, (Faber and Faber). In 1967 he was in many respects the architect or drafter of the bill otherwise known as the David Steel bill, which became the Abortion Act 1967. On the subject of the case of Alexandra he wrote to the *Times* arguing that (inter alia) it is wrong to compel parents of a severely handicapped infant to use the resources of modern medicine to prolong its life when they feel they cannot cope with it.

This argument is, with respect, wrong by omission. No one under present legislation can be forced to cope with children they do not want. Adoption and fostering have been discussed already. These options are always open to parents of severely handicapped infants.

Professor Williams argues the law should keep out of deciding such cases. He omits the point that the courts can be a useful arbiter and forgets their classic function of settling disputes.

His argument is that one who deliberately omits to save a life, that he is under a legal duty to save, is guilty of murder unless the law provides some defence. This omits much and is very misleading if left without qualification.

A doctor's duty is to act where permitted by law with reasonable skill, knowledge and care to try to save life (see Halsburys *Law of England*, 4th Edition para.34 & 35 etc.). The Geneva Convention states that doctors will maintain the utmost respect for human life from the time of conception. While it is possible that a parent having the power to save a child but who allowed it to drown might be charged with murder, nevertheless it is not clear that a doctor may or should perform surgical operations without the permission of the legal guardian under English law. Though in the case of the children of Jehovah's Witnesses, where blood transfusion is refused by the parents, the doctor may administer blood against the parents' wishes if he deems this to be a life saving act. There is considerable doubt in this area of the law and it is unfair to the medical profession to threaten as this letter continues to do that "On conviction of murder the penalty is a life sentence and the court has no discretion". The tone is more fitting for a hell-fire sermon. It drives a wedge between reality, which is that the law is there and must remain there to save lives at risk and the fiction that doctors will not do precisely that, in the overwhelming number of cases. It is also the law in wardship cases that the paramount interests of the child must be considered. The court has, therefore the capacity to allow a child to die where it would be officious to maintain it, but the right to life in so far as a general principle can be read from Alexandra's case, has been established.

As the *British Medical Journal* points out (29th August 1981), society needs to have principles and criteria in this heart-rending area. In reply to the statement that nature should be allowed to take its course in such a case as Alexandra it asks; "Do we want a society where fruitfulness determines the right to live?" The removal of the norm of sanctity of life plunges us all down the slippery slope into chaos and disagreement and is a further turning from what Christians believe that God wants, rich lives for all his children. But how is a rich life defined?

The importance of the sanctity of life view is that all are included under it; both parents and children, both deserve love and life. It is a theological not a legal principle. Professor Williams agrees in the introduction to his book (above) that these are sister professions. Callous regard has often been paid to life throughout history but little regard has often been paid to Christianity!

An injunction of Christ* is relevant to young, difficult children, "Do not despise one of these little ones!" Can we ignore this? Nor, as Christians, can we ignore the fact that God has a purpose for every child, which is beyond our understanding and He has a limitless ability to heal and comfort.

*Matthew 18:10.

13. CONCLUSION

Dr. Chandra Sethurajan

Medicine has made tremendous strides in alleviating many illnesses and eradicating others. Standards of health have improved almost worldwide. Life is improved for the disadvantaged by diligent application of knowledge and skill to meet specific needs. Continuing discoveries and advanced technology have influenced areas of human life hitherto outside the domain of man or science. This has created many new ethical and social challenges.

The medical profession has often been criticised for falling short of its social responsibilities. Professionalism it is said, has in some instances, made it difficult to provide positive help when needed. Many patients today feel they are becoming an object of study, research or a mere case number. Some trends in medical education are said to have moved the emphasis away from the patient. On the other hand, the evolution of team work in contemporary medical practice with due recognition being given to the role played by other paramedical disciplines and the members of the patient's family is genuinely progressive for patient care.

In this Year of the Disabled Person much exchange of useful information for self help, environmental aids and recreational activities designed for disabled people has taken place. Efforts have also been made to educate the public better, to become more sensitive to their needs.

These papers reaffirm our medical belief in the sanctity of life and so we have focussed on some contemporary issues, with ethical and social implications, that confront the medical profession.

Obviously there are other subjects which must be considered by those who are conscious of their social responsibility and not all have been dealt with in this book. To name a few, how has the recent trend of permissiveness and lack of personal discipline affected the lives of young people today? How can the stability of family life be secured for modern society? What are the missed opportunities in education? Where lie the new needs for Law Reform as the needs of society become increasingly pluralistic? In our time the world is threatened by nuclear explosion. Pollutants of all kinds threaten the earth. The finer values of life can be eroded unnoticed and destroy the fundamentals of a culture and its coherence in the name of change, progress or development.

Christ gave us two commandments. "You shall love the Lord your God with all your heart, with all your soul, with all your mind and with all your strength" and then "You shall love your neighbour as yourself."

To meet our neighbour's need we need the greatest use of our intelligence, all the knowledge and skill available. We also need all the sympathy and understanding possible for us and the creative aspiration that refuses to accept routine mediocrity. These need to be combined with all the practical help on any level that we can bring within the reach of those in need. Christian stewardship means the consecration of our whole personality to the service of God and so to man. To quote Archbishop Anthony Bloom,[1] "The prayer of the Church cannot ever be anything less than the prayer of Christ Himself. The spiritually alive live in a three dimensional world. Therefore we need to pray not only for ourselves but for our community, our nation and our world."

We hope that through these pages we have appealed to that "spark of divinity" that is in all of us so that readers are inspired to take a stand, find a vocation and look to a loving God for light in the darkness.

Notes

1.   Resident Archbishop of the Russian Orthodox Church in Great Britain.

SELECT BIBLIOGRAPHY

Catholic Truth Society. *Declaration on Euthanasia*, Sacred Congregation for the doctrine of the Faith, London 1980.

Chapman, J. A. and Goodall, J. "Helping a Child to Live Whilst Dying". *The Lancet* 5th April 1980.

Croshaw, T. *Killing Mercy?* International Pro-Life Information Centre, London.

General Synod Board for Social Responsibility. *On Dying Well*, GS 247, 1974.

Hinton, Professor J. "Dying". *Studies in Social Pathology*, Ed.C. Carstairs. Pelican Books, 1972.

Human Rights Society. *Human Value-or The Scrap Heap?* London, 1980.

Johnson, O.R. *Notes on Euthanasia*. Nationwide Festival of Light, London, 1975.

Koop, Dr. C. E. *The Right to Live, The Right to Die*. Tyndale, 1976.

Lamerton, Dr. R. *Care of the Dying*. Penguin, 1980.

Linacre Centre. *Reports 1–3. Prolongation of Life*, London 1978.

Macaulay, S. S. *Something Beautiful From God*. Marshall Morgan and Scott, London 1980.

Nilsson, L. *A Child is Born*. Faber Paperbacks, London, 1977.

O'Donovan, O. *The Christian and The Unborn Child*. Grove Books, Notts. 1973.

Rugg, M. D. and Carr, A. T. *Report to the Leicester Organisation For the Relief of Suffering*. Leicester 1976.

Schaffer, F. and Koop, Dr. C. E. *Whatever Happened To the Human Race?* Marshall, Morgan and Scott, London, 1979.

Society for the Protection of the Unborn Child. *Legal Abortion Examined*, A Human Concern Publication, London 1980.

Twycross, R. G. *The Dying Patient*. C.M.F. Publications, London 1975.

Willke, Dr. and Mrs J. C. *Handbook on Abortion*. Hayes Publishing Co. Inc., Ohio, USA.

Wilks, Professor E. *Terminal Care*. Report of working group chaired by Prof. Wilks, O.B.E. Sheffield 1980.

West, Dr. T. S. *Dictionary of Medical Ethics*. Contributions, "Attitude to Death", "Terminal Care" 1977 and 1981 Editions.

Zorza, Mr and Mrs V. *A Way to Die*. Andre Deutch, 1980.

Audio Visual Material

Death By Someone's Choice. A Series of three films. British Youth For Christ, Wolverhampton.

The Facts of Life. 37 slides with commentary, on the growth of the unborn, on abortion techniques and the work of LIFE.

I'd love to have her back though. A 41 minute 16mm film. Documentary on the life of the unborn as well as on abortion methods. Features Sir William Liley, 'father of foetology'. Order of Christian Unity. London.

The Story of Life. A 25 minute film (Both 8mm and 16mm). LIFE, Warwickshire.

THE AUTHORS

Sir John Peel—K.V.C.O., D.M., F.R.C.O.G., F.R.C.P., F.R.C.S

Past President Royal College of Obstetricians and Gynaecologists and of the British Medical Association. Hon. Consulting Obstetrician and Gynaecologist, King's College Hospital, and Hon. Fellow King's College Hospital Medical School.

Professor Ian Donald—C.B.E., M.D., F.R.C.O.G., F.R.C.S., Hon.F.A.C.O.G.

Regius Professor of Midwifery, University of Glasgow since 1954. Studied Medicine at St. Thomas's Hospital, graduating in 1937. MBE (Military Division) 1946. Reader in Obstetrics and Gynaecology St. Thomas's Hospital Medical School 1951. Reader, University of London, Institute of Obstetrics and Gynaecology, Hammersmith Hospital 1952. Eardley Holland Gold Medal from Royal College of Obstetricians and Gynaecologists 1970; Blair-Bell Gold Medal 1970, Royal Society of Medicine. Victor Bonney Prize, Royal College of Surgeons 1973. The McKenzie Davidson Medal 1975, British Institute of Radiology. At present Hon. Rottunda Consultant, National Maternity Hospital, Dublin. Hon. Obstetrician Western General Hospital, Edinburgh.

David D. C. Braine

David Braine at present Lecturer in Logic, University of Aberdeen, successively studied Physics, Modern History and finally Philosophy at Oxford between 1958–65, and since then has continued as lecturer in Logic and Metaphysics at the University of Aberdeen, publishing papers on philosophical, ethical and theological topics. In 1977, a spinal injury incurred as a passenger in a motor accident rendered him a paraplegic, which has occasioned some medical/paramedical teaching and writing in addition to his previous commitments.

Dr. Everett C. Koop M.D., Sc.D.(Med.)

At present Surgeon-General designate, U.S.A. After studying medicine at Cornell University, University of Pennsylvania and Eastern Baptist College, he has been Surgeon-in-Chief, Children's Hospital of Philadelphia since 1948. He was Editor-in-Chief *Journal of Pediatric Surgery* 1965–77 and is now a member of the British Association of Paediatric Surgeons from whom he received the Dennis Browne Gold Medal. He is also a member of the International Society of Surgery and a member of Paediatric Academies in France, Germany, Switzerland and the Dominican Republic. Publications include books and articles on surgery, biomedical ethics, physiology of the surgery of the neonate and technical advances in paediatric surgery.

Mrs. Patricia V. Seed, M.B.E., M.A.

Pat Seed is a journalist married to a Civil Engineer, has a son and a married daughter and two grandchildren.

She was diagnosed as having cancer in May 1976 and in January, 1977 the medical prognosis was that she could expect six months of life.

In March, 1977 she launched The Pat Seed Appeal Fund to provide the Christie Hospital with a CAT Scanner.

Mrs. Seed is now 53 years of age.

Mr. John Steensma

At present Head of the rehabilitation Department of Jackson Memorial Hospital, Miami, Florida.

Lost both arms (one above elbow, one below) at age of 17 by electrocution. Met future wife who persuaded him to enter College. Requested by U.S. Government to serve as amputee instructor during World War II in army hospital. Married, had four children. Directed program for amputees under World Council of Churches. Now Coordinator of Rehabilitation Center, University of Miami Medical Center, Florida.

Stuart J. Kingma, M.D.

At present Director of the Christian Medical Commission, World Council of Churches. Stuart Kingma was born in the USA and received his medical education at Cornell University Medical College in New York. He completed his surgical training at the Henry Ford Hospital in Detroit, and is a diplomat of the American Board of Surgery. He has worked with the Christian Medical Commission of the World Council of Churches since 1975, starting as Associate Director. Soon after his arrival, he assumed certain editorial responsibilities for The Commission's publication 'Contact' and has retained these up to the present.

Gordon Scorer, M.D., F.R.C.S.

Retired Consultant Surgeon, Hillingdon Hospital, Middlesex.

Dr. Thomas West, O.B.E. M.B., B.S.

At present, Deputy Medical Director, St. Christopher's Hospice. After qualifying at St. Thomas's Medical School Thomas West worked in various hospitals as House Surgeon until appointed Medical Superintendent of Wusasa Hospital in Nigeria, working with the Church Missionary Society. He was awarded the O.B.E. in 1972 for work in Nigeria., and appointed Visiting Consultant to the Hostel of God (now Trinity Hospice) in 1978. Apart from normal medical duties, he is responsible for organising the medical cover of the Hospice and is involved in a considerable number of outside lectures, both at home and abroad, to medical students, Post Graduate centres and groups interested in the care of the terminally ill. Publications include: 'The Final Voyage' *Frontier*, Vol 17 1974; 'Approach to death' *Nursing Mirror* 1974.

Group Captain Leonard Cheshire, V.C., D.S.O., D.F.C.

After studying Jurisprudence at Oxford, Leonard Cheshire had a distinguished career in the RAF, joining the British Joint Staff mission to Washington in 1945. He married Sue Ryder in 1959, and is the founder of the Cheshire Homes For the Disabled, which has 175 homes for disabled people in 35 countries. He is also co-founder of the Mission for the relief of Suffering, and in 1973 was awarded an honorary LLD by Liverpool University.

V. E. Hartley Booth, LL.B.(Bris), LL.B (Cantab), Dip. I.L.

Chairman of the Order of Christian Unity 1979–81. At present in practice at the bar, he has written *The Law of Extradition* and articles on other legal subjects. He has contributed to Bar Council Sub-Committee work and founded a voluntary organisation for the bedridden.

Dr. Chandra Sethurajan, M.B. B.S., D.C.H.(Lon.)

Has worked in London for the past ten years as Community Paediatrician in Hammersmith. She was born in Sri Lanka where she had a distinguished academic record, graduating in Medicine at the Christian Medical College, Vellore. After five years at various post graduate teaching hospitals in the U.K. and as an observer of the practice of Paediatrics in some European countries as well as the U.S. she returned as Paediatrician to the Women and Children's Mission Hospital in Inuvil, Sri Lanka for three years before returning to London. She is Chairman of the Order of Christian Unity Medical Committee.

THE MEDICAL COMMITEE

Sir John Peel, (Consultant)
Mr. V. E. Hartley Booth
Dr. Chandra Sethurajan, (Chairman)
Margaret Richards
Elizabeth Altwasser
Mr. Nigel Ruddock
Teresa Armstrong, (Editor)
Dr. Anne Booth
Dr. A. Harris

INDEX

Hippocratic Tradition, 2
Holt Radium Institute, Manchester, 35
Home-care programme, 75
Home Help Service, 74
Hospice Movement, 66–70; and home-care programme, 75; and pain
   control, 75–7
Housing, 75
Human life: value of, 6, 64–5; respect for, 68

Illegitimacy, 24; reduction of, 5
Illness, social and political factors in, 2; mental, 3, 73–4; diagnosis and
   treatment of, 7
Impairment, definition of, 44–5, 83
Inborn errors of metabolism, 14
Incontinence, 41, 73, 75
Incurable illness, 1, 5, 66–70
India, blind people in, 49
Information services, 29; need for, 51, 58
International Classification of Impairments, Disabilities and
   Handicaps, 44–5
International Year of Disabled Persons, 35, 44, 99
I.Q.: improvement in, in Down's Syndrome cases, 12–13, 92–3, 96

Jesus, healing ministry of, 63–4
Journal of the Royal Society of Medicine, 66

Kennedy, Ian, Reith Lectures, "Unmasking Medicine", 2, 6

Lane Report, 1974, 21
Law as arbitrator, 91, 96–8
Legislation, effects of, 6, 80–1, 99, 90–3
Leukaemia, 37
Life expectancy, 47
Life support system, withdrawal of, 73
Liley and Clarke, 14
Listening, as healing agent, 42
London Medical Group, 71
Love: 63; the international language, 36–8; as healing agent, 43

Malnutrition, and disability, 47, 55
Materialism in modern world, 2, 7, 27, 74
Medical Ethics, 1–2, 5, 6–7; Society for the Study of, 71
Medical profession, criticism of, 1, 6

Medicine: and behavioural problems, 3; curative, 4, 6; preventive, 4, 6; academic, 6; Christian dimension in, 63–4
Mental capacity, loss of, 73
Mental handicap, 5, 16–17; and genetic research, 11–12; and the family, 31
Mercy killing, 28–9, 64, 66–70, 90–1, 94; alternatives to, 66–70
Mongol Baby Case, 1981, 90–8
Mongolism. *See* Down's Syndrome.
Moral and ethical behaviour, 3
Mother Teresa of Calcutta, 64

National Health Service, financial problems of, 4
Nepal, incidence of blindness in, 49–50

Pain, control of, 66–7, 68, 71, 75–7, 78–9
Parens patriae, 93
Parents, role of, 13, 27–31, 90–1, 93–5, 96; rights of, 93
Patients, welfare of, 7, 99
Permissive trends, 1, 99; in legislation, 5
Pole, Hilary, 86
Poverty and disability, 50
Pregnancy, in schoolgirls, 1, 5
Preservation of Eyesight Project, 49
Prevention of disease, 2–3, 45–6, 49–50, 55–6
Progress v. traditional values, 1–2
Promiscuity, 5
Psychological factors in illness, 3, 20, 47

Rehabilitation, 27–8, 40–1, 47–50; western style, 58
Rehabilitation International, 50
Reith lectures. *See* Kennedy, Ian.
Religion, and medicine, 2
Resources, allocation of, 4, 6
Respect for life, 2, 67–8
Respiratory illness, 74
Responsible behaviour, 3
Responsible Society, the, 15
Resuscitation, 71, 73
Rh haemolytic disease, 14
Rubella in pregnancy, 13

St Christopher's Hospice, 66–70
St Teresa of Avila, 37–8
Sanctity of life, 64, 90, 96–8, 99